90 0943000 8

D1759815

WITHDRAWN FROM PL UNIVERSITY OF P

**Charles Seale-Hayne Library**
## University of Plymouth
**(01752) 588 588**
LibraryandITenquiries@plymouth.ac.uk

Feeling Bodies: Embodying Psychology

*Also by John Cromby*

PARENTAL INVOLVEMENT IN THE SEX EDUCATION OF STUDENTS WITH SEVERE LEARNING DIFFICULTIES: A Handbook (*with A. Craft*)

SOCIAL CONSTRUCTIONIST PSYCHOLOGY: A Critical Analysis of Theory and Practice (*edited with D.J. Nightingale*)

GLOBAL PERSPECTIVES ON THEORETICAL PSYCHOLOGY (*edited with P. Stenner, Y. He, J. Motzkau and J. Yen*)

PSYCHOLOGY, MENTAL HEALTH AND DISTRESS (*with D. Harper and P. Reavey*)

# Feeling Bodies: Embodying Psychology

John Cromby
*University of Leicester, UK*

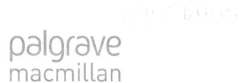

palgrave
macmillan

© John Cromby 2015

All rights reserved. No reproduction, copy or transmission of this publication may be made without written permission.

No portion of this publication may be reproduced, copied or transmitted save with written permission or in accordance with the provisions of the Copyright, Designs and Patents Act 1988, or under the terms of any licence permitting limited copying issued by the Copyright Licensing Agency, Saffron House, 6–10 Kirby Street, London EC1N 8TS.

Any person who does any unauthorized act in relation to this publication may be liable to criminal prosecution and civil claims for damages.

The author has asserted his right to be identified as the author of this work in accordance with the Copyright, Designs and Patents Act 1988.

First published 2015 by
PALGRAVE MACMILLAN

Palgrave Macmillan in the UK is an imprint of Macmillan Publishers Limited, registered in England, company number 785998, of Houndmills, Basingstoke, Hampshire RG21 6XS.

Palgrave Macmillan in the US is a division of St Martin's Press LLC, 175 Fifth Avenue, New York, NY 10010.

Palgrave Macmillan is the global academic imprint of the above companies and has companies and representatives throughout the world.

Palgrave® and Macmillan® are registered trademarks in the United States, the United Kingdom, Europe and other countries.

ISBN 978–1–137–38057–9

This book is printed on paper suitable for recycling and made from fully managed and sustained forest sources. Logging, pulping and manufacturing processes are expected to conform to the environmental regulations of the country of origin.

A catalogue record for this book is available from the British Library.

A catalog record for this book is available from the Library of Congress.

PLYMOUTH UNIVERSITY

9009470008

*David Smail (1938–2014) influenced me greatly, ever since I first read one of his books as an undergraduate. During the last decade or so of David's life, I was fortunate, with the other members of the Midlands Psychology Group, to work more closely with him. In doing so I benefited, not only from his reading, wisdom and courage, but from his dry wit and supremely eloquent swearing. It is with some justification that David was once described as 'psychology's Voltaire': this book is dedicated to him.*

# Contents

# Tables

# Acknowledgements

Towards the end of my PhD, my supervisor Penny Standen gave me a book about emotion. Her insightful gift prompted the interest that, eventually, led to this book.

In the lengthy course of writing this book, I have gained inspiration and support, both intellectual and practical, from many, many colleagues; I *feel* indebted to them all. Particular thanks must go to Steve Brown, Emma Chung, Tim Corcoran, Bob Diamond, Jan Soffe-Caswell, Kerry Chamberlain, Darren Ellis, Leanne Franklin, Dave Harper, Kieran O'Doherty, Paul Kelly, Antonia Lyons, Paul Moloney, Michael Murray, Dimitris Papadopoulos, Penny Priest, Peter Raggatt, Paula Reavey, John Shotter, Wendy Stainton-Rogers, Hank Stam, Paul Stenner, Thomas Teo, Chris Ward, Carla Willig and Martin Willis.

My mum and dad, and my friends and family, have been as consistently encouraging as ever. Special thanks to Karen for the cover image and to Rachel for pretty much everything. Thanks also to Liam for helping me to better understand the physics of sound, and much love – as always – to him and to Naomi, simply for being who they are.

The arguments in this book sometimes incorporate excerpts from previously published journal papers and book chapters. Specifically:

Thanks to Lawrence and Wishart for permission to use parts of 'Toward a Psychology of Feeling', originally published in the *International Journal of Critical Psychology*, 2007, 21: 94–118 (Chapters 1 and 4).

Thanks to Lawrence and Wishart for permission to use parts of 'Theorising Embodied Subjectivity', originally published in the *International Journal of Critical Psychology*, 2005, 15: 133–150 (Chapter 3).

Thanks to Taylor & Francis for permission to use parts of 'Affecting Qualitative Health Psychology', originally published in *Health Psychology Review*, 2011, 5: 79–96 (Chapter 5).

Thanks to John Wiley & Sons for permission to use parts of 'The Greatest Gift: Happiness, Governance and Psychology', originally published in *Social and Personality Psychology Compass*, 2011, 5, 11: 840–852 (Chapter 5).

Thanks to Sage Publications for permission to use parts of 'Beyond Belief' and 'Responses to Commentaries on "Beyond Belief"', originally published in the *Journal of Health Psychology*, 2012, 17, 7: 943–957 and 17, 7: 982–987 (Chapter 6).

Thanks to Sage Publications and to Dr Dave Harper for permission to use parts of 'Paranoia: A Social Account', published in *Theory & Psychology*, 2009, 19, 3: 335–361 (Chapter 8).

Thanks to Professor Chris Ward for permission to reuse parts of 'Public Meanings of CFS/ME: Making Up People', originally published in *Meanings of ME: Interpersonal and Social Dimensions of Chronic Fatigue* (2015) London, Palgrave (Chapter 7).

Thanks to Dr Alastair Morgan for permission to reuse parts of 'Feelings, Beliefs and Being Human', originally published in *Being Human: Reflections on Mental Distress in Society* (2008) Ross-on-Wye, PCCS Books (Chapter 8).

# 1
# Introducing

Before we are anything else, we are feeling bodies. Feelings – novel, satisfying, intense, prolonged, challenging or transcendent – are sought by bungee jumpers, mountaineers and practitioners of 'extreme' sports; by millions of consumers of alcohol, tobacco, caffeine and other recreational drugs; by users of pornography, music and painkillers; and by consumers at festivals, carnivals, fairgrounds, music events, cinemas and sports stadia. The management of feeling is integral to identities that are both gendered ('big boys don't cry') and cultural ('keep a stiff upper lip') and emphasised by advice to 'keep a cool head' to make unbiased, rational decisions. Simultaneously, the fabric of everyday relating includes countless conversations that begin with some reference to feeling ("So, how are you today?"), conversations of which a sizeable minority take feeling as their primary focus ("I'm sorry I upset you"). In fact, the ubiquity and relevance of feeling is such that sometimes it is even parodied ("so – how does that make you *feel?*").

Viewed from the perspective of the public realm, feelings are the target for manipulation and inculcation in advertising, propaganda, public relations and politics: from the crowd manipulation techniques developed by Goebbels to multinational corporations' use of phenomena such as the mere exposure effect (Zajonc, 1980) and attempts to associate positive feelings with brands in order to foster loyalty (Barsky & Nash, 2002); or politicians' use of contrasts and three-part lists to generate approval (Atkinson, 1984), and 'dog-whistle' phrases to mobilise support (Goodin & Saward, 2005). Recently, there has been greatly increased interest in feelings within social science and humanities disciplines, including sociology, cultural studies, geography, criminology, economics and history, as well as within psychology. And feelings – specifically, of happiness and well-being – have even emerged as a goal

1

of UK government policy, with the creation of a new national index purporting to provide an assessment of their demographic associations and annual movements (Cromby, 2011).

## Troubling concepts

But what are feelings? For now it is enough to think of feelings as bodily states that can be subjectively experienced. Understood this way, feelings are not just emotions, although they include components of emotion. Hunger, thirst, tiredness, itchiness and pain are all feelings, despite their typical characterisation in psychology as mere sensations (a category seen at once as more primitive than the cognitions presumed to dominate them). Feelings also include the heterogeneous somatic experiences associated with moods and inclinations, and the vague, fluctuating, liminal states associated with as-yet tentative desires, or with emergent judgements that an argument, claim or situation *feels* either right or wrong (feelings that bear no necessary relation to more intersubjective criteria of truth and accuracy).

It is nevertheless notoriously difficult to identify consistently agreed definitions of feeling, affect, emotion and related terms. This is in part because the phenomena they index are known in their fullness only subjectively or experientially and are therefore, to some extent, private. Simultaneously, important components of these phenomena are embodied and therefore somewhat *ineffable* (Stam, 1998; Shilling, 2003): not capable of being wholly represented using words or symbols. Moreover, at the same time, it seems to be a characteristic of feelings that they have us before we have them. Feeling arises within experience without our needing to reflect upon it – however much its appearance then demands reflection, and however much that subsequent reflection is shaped and constituted by the intensities and preoccupations it brings.

Feeling is thoroughly embedded in history, and this extends to the basic concepts that designate it. Whilst in the (not too-distant) past we might have discussed passions, appetites, sentiments, affections and sensibilities, today we talk about emotions, moods, affects and feelings. And just as feeling is embedded in history, so it is also infused with culture. There are culture-specific emotions such as *toska*: a Russian term for an experience blended from what Anglo-Americans see as two relatively distinct emotions – anxiety or fear, and sadness (Ogarkova et al., 2012). Conversely, it is often claimed that, for good evolutionary reasons, 'disgust' is a culturally universal emotion. However, Wierzbicka (1999) notes that in Polish there is no word that corresponds exactly to this English term – a peculiar state of affairs if disgust, conceived in Anglo-American terms as a specific and distinct affective capacity,[1] really were universal. Wierzbicka also describes how Polish people experience an emotion, *tesknota*, which has parallels with homesickness and nostalgia, and with experiences of missing someone or 'pining' for them, yet which differs from each of these. Other likely examples of culture-specific emotions include *amae, schadenfreude* and *amok*.

More fundamentally, the very notion of the affective as a distinct realm separable from the cognitive is perhaps itself a cultural construction. Lutz (1988) describes how the Ifaluk of Papua New Guinea have no concepts that correspond to the categories of thought and emotion. Their term, *nunuwan*, which translates roughly as 'being' or 'experience', uniformly encompasses all of the phenomena that Anglo-Americans typically parse into these two distinct categories. Ifaluk people do experience what we would call emotions, moods or feelings, but they do not understand these experiences as belonging to a category that is distinguishable from another containing other experiences called 'thoughts'. Consequently, whereas Anglo-Americans see maturation from childhood as involving a process of learning to regulate, tame or control emotion, the Ifaluk see it as one of increasing and differentiating *nunuwan*. And, as Ratner (2000) notes, there are other cultures such as the Illongot who do not sharply distinguish the cognitive from the affective.

So affective phenomena are intimate, experiential and embodied, incapable of perfect capture or absolute representation in language, yet, at the same time, thoroughly bound up with and shaped by history and culture. So perhaps it is not surprising that they seem constantly to elude singular and agreed definitions, or, more accurately, that they appear capable of accommodating multiple yet somewhat incompatible conceptualisations. It is similarly unsurprising that these concepts mutate over time and travel imperfectly between cultures, notwithstanding that there must be elements of the affective that, just like the human capacity for language, are endowed by our species-nature.

Despite this, psychology predominantly treats concepts of affect, emotion and feeling as largely unproblematic. In psychology, the cognitive contains elements such as words, symbols, factual knowledge, beliefs and attitudes, and processes such as attention, memory encoding and recall, learning, judging, reasoning, calculating, problem solving and decision-making. The affective, by contrast, contains emotions such as happiness, sadness, surprise, anger, fear, disgust, shame, guilt and so on. It also contains moods, which like emotions are valenced and have motivational effects, but which differ from them in being both less focused (their cause or object is often unclear) and more temporally extended. Feeling is also typically included within the affective, where it is sometimes a synonym for emotion, sometimes used to refer specifically to emotions' phenomenological aspects ('he felt angry'), but sometimes also recruited into cognitive analyses (e.g. in research into the 'tip of the tongue' phenomena).

Nevertheless, this does not mean that psychology has a single, agreed concept of emotion. And indeed, psychology is not the only relevant discipline to be characterised by such multiplicity. In her introductory text on emotion science, a field informed by psychology, neuroscience and other disciplines, Fox (2008, p. 23) frankly acknowledges that "there is no general agreement in emotion science on how emotion should be defined".

For example, despite being the target of numerous well-founded critiques, some research still invokes the notion of basic emotions. This is the idea that a core set of emotions – most commonly anger, sadness, surprise, happiness, disgust and fear (Ekman, 1992) – are universal within our species. These emotions are said to be enabled by genetically endowed, hardwired neural modules, the existence of which can, at least in principle, be associated with selection pressures flowing from the survival or reproductive advantages produced by the action potentials and states of preparedness that these capacities bestowed: to fight off predators (anger), manage changes in social status (sadness), prepare for something unexpected (surprise), cement a social bond (happiness), avoid something toxic (disgust) or retreat from something dangerous (fear).

The most influential current conceptualisation of emotion is probably Scherer's (e.g. 2009a) component process theory. Here, emotions are complex phenomena that simultaneously recruit cognitive and somatic capacities in orchestrated patterns where multiple levels and components of information processing combine to appraise situations and prepare individuals, mentally and physically, for appropriate action. There are five core components in Scherer's model: cognitive (appraisal), neurophysiological (bodily), motivational (action tendencies), motor expression (facial and vocal) and subjective feeling. These combine in dynamic, variable patterns, constituted of multiple feedback loops and bidirectional influences, to generate central representations of brain–body states to which verbal categorisations and labels (e.g. 'angry') get added; this representation and labelling then loops back into the appraisal processes that began the entire cascade.

Another prominent notion of emotion is supplied by core affect theory (Barrett, 2006), where physiological changes in valence states and arousal levels combine with stored representations (shaped, amongst other influences, by culture) to generate different emotional experiences. But there are also other concepts of emotion, including notions derived from psychoanalysis and its variants such as attachment theory, along with more recent conceptualisations such as that proffered by discursive psychology, which treats emotion as an interactional resource and accomplishment (Edwards, 1999).

In the social sciences and humanities, where what is being called an 'affective turn' has been occurring (e.g. Blackman & Cromby, 2007; Clough & Halley, 2007; Athanasiou, Hantzaroula, & Yannakopoulos, 2008; Blackman, 2012), parallel diversity is evident and at least three distinct concepts of affect have been influential. The first is Tompkins' affect theory, an early variant of basic emotion theory which strongly emphasised the ways in which affect can flow in complex, recursive circuits and feedback loops both within and between individuals. Tompkins' theory has been taken up by writers such as Probyn (2004) and Sedgewick and Frank (1995) within their penetrating analyses of shame. The second comes from psychoanalysis, where affect refers to primary-process activity, the seething motives, nameless compulsions and unspeakable desires of the unconscious, the operations of which are forever too threatening to be known directly and so must always be diluted or disguised before they enter awareness (Mitchell & Black, 1995). The third and the most influential conception of affect comes from the work of Deleuze and Guattari, and specifically through its interpretation by Massumi (2002). Here, affect is the capacity of organisms to act upon and be acted upon by their worlds,[2] a capacity that is both interpellated ('called out') and impelling. Affect is pre-personal, before experience and consisting of 'unqualified intensities' that constitute and precede the sociolinguistic. Unlike its 'captured' residue, emotion, affect is an untamed force, neither individual nor specifically human, but a general property of living things and the motive force for becoming – the ceaseless process of restless change that characterises life itself.

When conceptual clarity is needed but the empirical evidence is ambiguous, philosophical analysis may help. Philosophers often equate affect with irrationality and contrast it against calm, rational judgement, treating emotion and feeling as something to be managed and regulated so that neutral, calm judgements can be made. Hence Aristotle recommended moderation with respect to emotion, whereas the Stoics advocated rigorous control. Nevertheless, philosophers also disagree about the limits and character of the affective. Spinoza saw affect as a fundamental power of the body, a notion that reappears in Deleuze's work. Hume saw reason as the "slave of the passions", treating their dominance as not only inevitable but also morally or normatively correct. Recent work by Griffiths (1998) grapples more directly with the character of emotions, proposing that they lie on a continuum from basic to culture-specific – effectively, from the wholly biological to the wholly socially constructed – with an in-between region occupied by what he calls 'higher cognitive emotions' not unique to particular cultures and containing marked cognitive components. By contrast, Prinz (2004) argues that no emotion is wholly biological since, to be understood and recognised, it must necessarily have a cultural aspect: at least in a weak sense, all emotions are socially constructed (Harre, 1986). But simultaneously, no emotion is *wholly* socially constructed, since all experience is also necessarily embodied. Hence *all* emotions occupy something like the middle ground that Griffiths identifies – although Prinz's characterisation of them as 'embodied appraisals' subverts the emphasis that Griffiths places upon cognitive factors.

### Feeling the way

Ultimately then, neither psychology nor any other field seems able to decide exactly what the affective realm contains, nor agree precisely where its boundaries lie. This has implications across the discipline because many psychological concepts, usually treated or described as simply cognitive, actually straddle the presumed cognition–affect divide. For example, self-esteem contains a prominent affective dimension, alongside or bound up with its representational, discursive or cognitive elements (Scheff & Fearon, 2004). And, as I will argue later, the psychological concept of belief can also be considered as such a hybrid. Nevertheless, it is not that we don't know anything about affect, emotion and feeling. At the same time, what we do know lacks coherence, and – despite frequent claims in psychology to be strictly empirical or 'scientific' – rests (if only because of the methodologies deployed) upon implicit assumptions that are culturally and historically specific.

In this book, I will navigate through this uncertainty by consistently emphasising feeling, in preference to affect or emotion. The intention is not to institute a sharp definitional distinction between the three terms, but to develop an argument that feeling is integral to the phenomena described by each of them. Hence I will sometimes use adjectives such as 'affective' to refer to the realm of embodied influence and responsiveness within which what get called affect, emotion and feeling are significant, whilst still favouring feeling as a central concept. This preference is partly because, unlike affect and emotion, 'feeling' is a linguistic prime: all human cultures, so far as we know, have a word or concept that denotes feeling (Shweder, 2004), making it a strong candidate upon which to base analysis. The term also emphasises the psychological, whilst potentially sidestepping some of the uncertainty surrounding definitions of emotion and affect. It largely (although not exclusively) ties analysis to the experiential realm, and in this way might constrain some of the 'overspill' or indeterminacy that Wetherell (2012) associates with analyses of affect. This is in part because, unlike contemporary notions of affect, the concept of feeling elaborated here does not reside "outside social meaning" (Hemmings, 2005, p. 565): consequently, it might avoid some of the problems noted by Hemmings, Wetherell and others (e.g. Leys, 2011).[3] Finally, feeling is a more inclusive concept than affect or emotion, potentially encompassing a considerably broader range of bodily states and experiences. This makes feeling especially valuable for analyses of health and illness, such as those presented later, because – alongside the emotional – feeling includes the sensations associated with pain, fatigue and other relevant bodily experiences.

## Embodying psychology

A central argument of this book is that a focus upon feelings might facilitate an embodied psychology: one that takes seriously the observation that absolutely all experience depends upon our living bodies for its very character, as well as its mere possibility (Merleau-Ponty, 2002). But emphasising the living body also means challenging the successive mechanical metaphors that have dominated psychology, metaphors Leary (1994) traces back to Descartes' separation of the immaterial soul from the material body-machine it was said to temporarily inhabit. Freudian psychoanalysis, for example, invokes a hydraulic metaphor: Victorian steam-driven machinery supplied a model of mind pushed by hidden forces, a mind which must regulate, balance and control the seething pressures that provide its impetus. Behaviourist psychology, by contrast, emphasised external quasi-mechanical functions. Subjective capacities such as feeling, even if their occurrence could be reliably demonstrated, were treated as epiphenomenal: the study of behaviour did not require any consideration of experience. Byrne (1994) uses the analogy of a clock, the hands of which produce 'time-telling behaviour'. Under behaviourism, the clock's inner workings – water-driven, spring-coiled, battery-operated, solar-powered, pendulum-regulated, radio-controlled – were ignored: what mattered was understanding the patterns in which its hands moved. Researchers explored how different reinforcement schedules caused organisms (much data was gathered using rats, pigeons, dogs and other animals) to produce altered response patterns. Their experiments positioned living creatures as appendages to the machines that conditioned them – to press levers, push buttons, solve mazes, salivate, startle, blink and so on.

More recently, psychology has been dominated by a computational metaphor where functions and abilities are understood largely in terms of information processing. Impelled to a notable extent by covert military funding (Bowers, 1990), the so-called cognitive revolution contributed to an interdisciplinary effort to reproduce in machines the advanced cognitive abilities of humans, by developing and testing computer models of human capacities.[4] The computer metaphor yields a psychology that closely resembles the head on this book's cover, in that it is for the most part individual, lifeless, artificial and disembodied. Other metaphors also inform cognitive psychological research: in relation to memory alone, Hoffman, Cochran and Nead (1990) list metaphors including a wax tablet, house full of rooms, dictionary, encyclopaedia, muscle, telephone switchboard, computer, hologram, conveyor belt or archaeological reconstruction. Nonetheless, these other metaphors are consistently subordinated to an overarching computational notion of information processing, a presumed general cognitive ability that might equally be enabled by silicon and wire as by flesh and blood.

Shotter (1993, p. 153) observes that one of the first tasks facing students of psychology is to "begin by treating such terms (as 'computer', 'information processor' or 'mind') as representing real objects which are at first only vaguely known to them". He suggests that the initial difficulty and strangeness of this task reveals how cognitive psychology can be considered, in Foucauldian terms, as a discursive regime working to bind researchers into groups, all ostensibly studying the same object. Within this regime, well-known tropes such as the Turing test do important work of establishing the primacy of cognition and information processing – albeit that "it is only possible to 'see' a similar logic in the activities of computers (or information processing systems) and people, if we agree at the outset to ignore everything to do with their different material instantiation" (op. cit., p. 155).

Like computers themselves, the computational metaphor is a complex, flexible one that potentially includes networks and hardware as well as software and information. This means that the growing influence of neuroscience is being incorporated into psychology, at least thus far, without any overall substitution of this dominant metaphor. Information processing requires algorithms to arrange its processes – software – and computers upon which those algorithms can run: hardware. Cognitive psychology has tended to emphasise these algorithms, producing what are effectively software models of memory formation, memory retrieval, selective attention and such like. Whilst neuroscience is shifting the focus from software towards hardware – the brain structures and neural networks that enable information processing – the prevailing computational metaphor is largely being retained. In the words of Professor Ray Dolan, speaking of the inauguration of the UCL Computational Psychiatry centre, "The brain is at some level an information processing machine and we have to understand what it's doing and how that information processor is working" (Siddique, 2014).

The influence of this metaphor is apparent even in relation to emotion. Scherer's component process model of emotion is frequently represented as a flowchart; he has written of its consonance with computer modelling of human behaviour (Scherer, 2009b); and he typically presents the model using computational language. However, psychologists have long recognised that mechanical metaphors of emotion are unhelpful. Discussing mental health problems and treatments, Smail (1984) contrasted the 'debug the software' approach of cognitive therapy with the 'mend the hardware' strategy of psychiatric drug treatments. He argued that, in depending upon the same computational metaphor, both approaches are falsely optimistic. They potentially mislead both practitioners and service users into imagining that interventions could utterly transform emotionally distressed people into others, for whom it were as though distress had never actually occurred. Rejecting this cruelly false hope, Smail instead proposed an organic metaphor by comparing the person to a tree once hit by a vehicle. If we examine the rings of the tree, the large dent when the vehicle initially struck will get continuously smaller with each successive year's growth. However, the impact will always remain part of its structure, and the tree hit by a vehicle will always differ somewhat from its neighbour that escaped collision.

The philosopher Susanne Langer (whose work will be a frequent resource in this book) suggests that mechanical metaphors will always mislead precisely because humans are living creatures, not machines. From its inception, psychology failed to adequately consider the profound differences between the living and the mechanical, in part due to its Cartesian heritage, and also because it rapidly adopted methods and procedures from physics (whilst also borrowing a swathe of concepts, largely unreflexively, from the folk psychology of everyday life). In this way, the nascent discipline missed out a vital "state of having turbulent notions about things that seem to belong together, although in some unknown way...a prescientific state, a sort of intellectual gestation period" (Langer, 1967, p. 52). During this time, psychology might have formulated "different ideas, different expectations, without concern for experiments or statistics or formalised language" (op. cit.). This fertile period might have allowed psychologists to generate a rich conceptual framework adequate to their subject matter that would foster sound hypotheses and appropriate methods, so creating a robust discipline within which "experiments should suggest themselves automatically, and techniques and language grow up apace" (op. cit.). But psychology missed this phase as the discipline rapidly oriented itself towards pragmatic solutions for contemporary social issues, and this orientation, reciprocally, shaped its methods and concepts (Danziger, 1994).

Rejecting mechanical metaphors does not mean rejecting the systematic development of psychological knowledge. It means recognising that, fundamentally, psychology is an organismic process and not a computational or mechanical activity. To understand it, we must therefore develop concepts and methods that engage with the concrete specificities of organic, felt experience – even if this leads to the conclusion that "the study of mental and social phenomena will never be 'natural science' in the familiar sense at all, but will always be more akin to history, which is a highly codified discipline, but not an abstractly codified one" (Langer, 1967, p. 53).

## Neuroscience

The proposal that psychology should consider the organic processes enabling experience leads, almost inevitably in the present moment, to neuroscience, and this presents something of a dilemma. On the one hand, it is impossible to ignore: a book on the embodiment of psychology that did not consider any evidence from contemporary neuroscience would lack plausibility. On the other hand, there are various problems associated both with the evidence from neuroscience and with its typical interpretations.

Much of the evidence flows from imaging research using scanning techniques such as magnetic resonance imaging (MRI), positron emission tomography (PET) and magnetoencephalography (MEG). A great many studies use functional MRI (fMRI) techniques which model differential patterns of local brain activation, producing highly coloured graphics that seemingly picture the living brain in the very process of thinking. Cautioning against such simplistic interpretations, Rose and Abi-Rachid (2013) first of all note that naïve claims of localisation are usually premature since most neural tasks involve distributed networks joining many areas. Suggestions that neuroscientists have found 'the part of the brain for' an activity almost invariably ignore how brains function as massively networked, massively parallel ensembles. They also urge critical consideration of the scale upon which localisation is postulated, quoting an analysis which shows that in fMRI a typical voxel (the basic unit of comparison) contains as many as 5.5 million neurons with "between $2.2 \times 10^5$ and $5.5 \times 10^{10}$ synapses, 22 km of dendrites and 220 km of axons" (Rose & Abi-Rachid, 2013, p. 76).

The temporal resolution of fMRI is also quite limited. Measurable changes in local blood-oxygen levels (upon which fMRI scanning depends) arise relatively slowly and can only be accurately detected down to about one second. By contrast, elementary processes such as transferring visual signals from the retina to the thalamus and visual cortex require only tens of milliseconds. Whilst some other processes may take longer, they are still measured in very small fractions of a second – and, famously, even half a second is a long time in brain terms (Libet, 1993).

Rose and Abi-Rachid (2013) also describe how imaging studies treat the laboratory, and the various processes by which participants are inducted and managed within experiments, as neutral and lacking impact. In fact, they are patently social settings and interactions that necessarily have consequences for participants. Following Joseph Dumit (2004), they describe how there are actually four stages involved in the production of imaging data:

1 developing the research design, choosing participants and control groups, choosing a task
2 managing the technical process, conducting scans, compiling data, using algorithms to construct three-dimensional models
3 making the data comparable, combining images and warping them onto a standardised brain anatomical atlas
4 making the data presentable, using specialist software packages to introduce colour and contrast and generate high quality images (p.78).

Each stage of this process implicates many assumptions – about the research topics, the participants' capabilities, the significances of the BOLD (blood-oxygen level dependent) signal which fMRI detects and how all these relate to the functions of the living brain and the tasks that participants completed. Additionally, the algorithms and software packages utilised rest upon a further series of complex mathematical assumptions that also influence what the study will reveal, but the nature and implications of those assumptions remain largely invisible. Other scholars have also raised cautionary points. Cacioppo et al. (2003) describe how the 'subtraction method' used in many studies involves comparing average levels of activation in different brain regions between participants in both experimental (task) and control (resting) conditions, effectively by subtracting one from the other. They observe that, by itself, the method neither demonstrates that activation of specific brain regions shows that they *are* functionally necessarily for a task, nor that absence of activation shows that they are not. They also show how this method produces findings based upon average patterns that might not have actually been observed in any study participant, and conversely, how it can make areas that are continuously active appear irrelevant. Discussing the application of neuroscience to psychotherapy, Manteufel (2005) observes that most imaging studies simply correlate patterns of brain activation with some task, activity or event, and that this leaves many of the most interesting questions – for example, whether the activity was excitatory or inhibitory – unanswered. Relatedly, I have argued that the typical design of imaging studies makes them ecologically invalid and involves a practice of methodological individualism that empirically precludes many of the emergent properties of naturally occurring groups and collectives that we might wish to understand (Cromby, 2007).

Importantly, none of these analyses suggest that we simply dismiss brain-imaging studies; rather that we interpret them far more critically and cautiously. Rose and Abi-Rachid propose that we begin by rejecting the 'photographic illusion' of objectivity they create. Brain scanning produces graphic representations of computer models of brain activity (or, more precisely, of regional variations in blood-oxygen levels), but these graphics are simulations – not photographs. They do not *picture* what the brain was doing; they *model* what the data – and the many assumptions upon which it rests – suggests that it might have been doing.

Whilst this shift of interpretation would help neutralise naïve interpretations of neuroscientific research, deeper problems remain. As Tallis

(2009) wryly observes, neuroscience "reveals some of the most impor-tant conditions that are *necessary* for behaviour and awareness" but does not "provide a satisfactory account of the conditions that are *sufficient*". In a similar vein, Harre (2002) carefully distinguishes between enabling and causing: our brains and bodies make possible – enable – every expe-rience we ever have – but this does not mean they simply *cause* those experiences. Nevertheless, interpretations of imaging studies often pro-ceed as though the brain activity is simply equivalent to the activity of thinking, as though neural activity and phenomenological experience were essentially identical.

At stake here is the so-called 'hard problem' of how physical pro-cesses in the body and brain can give rise to conscious experiences (Chalmers, 1995). A collaborative analysis between a neuroscientist and a philosopher (Bennett & Hacker, 2003) shows how in neuroscience this problem is frequently managed (in the sense of being concealed or bypassed, rather than solved) by simply treating the mind as though it were equivalent to the brain. They call this tendency a mutant or degenerate form of Cartesian dualism. Whereas Cartesian thinking asso-ciated psychological processes (believing, choosing, deciding, etc.) with the mind, contemporary neuroscience often simply associates them with the brain. They argue that both are mistaken since these pro-cesses can logically only be attributed to persons, not to their isolated parts:

> It is not that as a matter of fact brains do not think, hypothesise and decide, see and hear, ask and answer questions; rather, it makes no sense to ascribe such predicates *or their negations* to the brain. The brain neither sees, *nor is it blind* – just as sticks and stones are not awake, *but they are not asleep either*. The brain does not hear, but it is not deaf, any more than trees are deaf. The brain makes no decisions, but nor is it indecisive. Only what *can* decide can be indecisive. So, too, the brain cannot be conscious; only the living creature whose brain it is can be conscious – or unconscious. *The brain is not a logically appropriate subject for psychological predicates.*
>
> (Bennett & Hacker, 2003, p. 72, emphases in original)

Bennett and Hacker also demonstrate how there will always be limits to what can be discovered using neuroscientific experimental procedures. Using the example of writing a signature, they argue that even if we knew considerably more about the many brain processes involved in its production – perhaps, even, if we could measure *everything* that was happening in the brain as the signature was written – a comprehensive explanation would still elude us since

> no amount of neural knowledge would suffice to discriminate between writing one's name, copying one's name, practising one's signature, forging a name, writing an autograph, signing a cheque, witnessing a will, signing a death warrant, and so on...the differences between these are circumstance-dependent, functions not only of the individual's intentions but also of the social and legal conventions that must obtain to make the having of such intentions and the performance of such actions possible.
>
> (Bennett & Hacker, 2003, p. 360)

So brain-imaging studies produce graphic simulations, not pictures, and these are at a considerably greater scale – both spatial and temporal – than that at which actual brain activity occurs. The assumptions and practices of experimentation influence what these studies show, as do the assumptions necessarily embedded in the analysis of data. At the same time, the findings of experiments can only ever be interpreted in relation to social and cultural contexts that their procedures do not include. Moreover, these interpretations frequently gloss over the profound difference between neural activity and psychological experience.

Whilst neuroscience also includes findings from lesion studies, neuroanatomy, electroencephalography and animal research, as well as from other imaging techniques, these methods have their own limitations (some of which they share with brain imaging, and others which are more particular). Moreover, as the preceding discussion demonstrates, the difficulties are not merely methodological or empirical – more profoundly, they are also conceptual. Consequently, in this book, I will acknowledge that neuroscience undoubtedly tells us something about how brain and body are related, as well as how they might enable feeling. But I will also assume that it is possible to question the findings of many experiments, which must often be considered provisional, partial and sensitively dependent upon their specific conditions of production. Where I engage with neuroscience, it will therefore be in a particular fashion. Rather than cite and interpret single studies, I will typically consider broad patterns of findings – for example, to do with the general pattern of relations between processes described as cognitive and those described as affective. In practice, this will often mean attending equally to books, review articles and opinion pieces by neuroscientists and other scholars, as well as to the studies these writings discuss. Also, neuroscience will largely be used in an illustrative rather than a foundational manner: it will not be ignored, but neither will strong claims be made on the basis of its evidence alone. The topic of this book is psychology, not neuroscience, and the primary interest is feeling rather than the neural substrates that enable it. Whilst neuroscience is relevant to this endeavour, it supplies only one part of the picture.

## Situating psychology

In addition to arguing that a focus on feeling might produce an embodied psychology, this book will also argue that most feelings are both socialised – shaped by prior experience – and social, responsive to aspects of the present moment. Yet, feeling so intimately saturates who and how we are that it can feel strange, even threatening, to argue that it is social at the very same time as it is individual. This tendency might be particularly pronounced in cultures such as ours,[5] which promote relatively sharp distinctions between individuals and their material and social environments. We are frequently encouraged to see ourselves as standing out against our social relations, rather than continuously embedded within and shaped by them; to see ourselves as overcoming or controlling our environments, rather than recognising how our activities are continuously enabled by them. Consequently, we tend to imagine ourselves largely independent and self-sufficient, rather than appreciating how our freedoms to act and decide are always produced and sustained by the diverse ways in which they are already embedded in relays and networks of socio-culturally shaped relationships and resources.

These cultural tendencies towards individualism are frequently mirrored and amplified by ideological forces which emphasise self-sufficiency, moral autonomy and personal responsibility. Sometimes collectively described as neoliberalism, these ideological tendencies are currently dominant in many countries. They are associated with growing social inequality, the scaling back and withdrawal of health, education and social care, and a concomitant emphasis on choice and individual obligation (Brown, 2006; Fyson & Cromby, 2013).

This combination of cultural tendencies and ideological influences will be further intensified, for many readers of this book, by their training in a psychology which had its primary focus upon the individual. This focus differentiates psychology from the more overtly social disciplines such as sociology, anthropology, economics, politics, social policy and cultural studies. It also differentiates psychology from disciplines such as neuroscience, anatomy and physiology which emphasise parts of, and biological processes within, bodies. It means that psychology is constantly pulled in different directions: towards the social in one direction, towards the biological in the other and towards what seems to be pure thought – cognition – in the virtual space between (a space manifested by another cultural tendency, that towards Cartesian or mind–body dualism).

We see these pulls reflected in the way psychology divides into relatively distinct sub-disciplines: social psychology, cognitive psychology, biological psychology and so on. This fracturing seemingly enables psychology to embrace both the biological and the social aspects of experience, and occasionally even to unite or integrate them. In practice, however, biological psychology is largely separate from cognitive psychology, which in turn is largely separate from social psychology. Researchers within each sub-discipline mostly publish in different journals, attend different conferences, pose different research questions and pursue different funding streams.

It will always be necessary to organise psychological knowledge, research and teaching in some way or other. Yet, its current organisation has the peculiar consequence that psychology is held together by an illusion. Psychology emphasises individuals, rather than the cultures and groups of which they are part, or the biological processes by which both individuality and collectivity are sustained. But the individual produced by cognitive psychology – which typically looks something like a flowchart or computer program – fundamentally differs from the individual produced by biological psychology, which typically looks something like a brain or part thereof. Both differ from the individual produced by social psychology, which is enmeshed within groups or collectives and consequently has more explicitly permeable boundaries. And each of these differs again from the self-actualising individual of humanistic psychology, the covertly depraved individual of Freudian psychoanalysis, or the positive psychological individual for whom selfhood is an endless (and frankly unfeasible) DIY project.

Ultimately, then, psychology's focus on the individual is an illusion because there is no consensus with regard to what an individual is. The psychological individual is a boundary object or a black box[6] (Robertson, 2001) that allows the sub-disciplines to hang (somewhat gingerly) together, thereby facilitating the institutional management of research and teaching. And this works, after a fashion, provided no one opens the box to see what is inside.

So a combination of qualities, forces and habits of thought combine to encourage a view of feelings as wholly private and individual. First, their ubiquitous character and their capacity to intimately suffuse experience can make them seem both precious and unique. Second, cultural tendencies towards individualism reinforce the notion that we are self-contained, isolated monads for whom society and culture are contexts but not, to any serious extent, constituents. Third, there are ideological tendencies, reinforced and made real – reified – by associated societal institutions and practices. And fourth, psychology is held together by an *illusion* of the individual, and awareness of this amongst the more thoughtful might itself impel defensive tendencies to reassert individualism.

## This book

This book describes how feeling occupies a liminal space: between mind and body, and strung out between self and others; of each, yet reducible to none. It is constituted through history, culture, social relations and materiality, at the very same time that it is subjectively experienced by individuals in the sensuous intimacy of their living flesh. Because of these characteristics, feeling has considerable potential to supply the basis of a psychology that is at once living, organic and situated, rather than static, mechanical and abstract.[7]

The structure of the book is relatively straightforward. In Chapter 2, 'Feeling', Susanne Langer's concept of feeling and its primordially constitutive relationship with experience is described. Analytical distinctions between different types of feeling are explained, relevant terminologies are identified and there is a sustained focus upon how feeling continuously constitutes experience whilst simultaneously tending to recede into the background of activity.

Whilst Langer's notion of feeling has much to commend it, overall she pays insufficient attention to the social realm. Chapter 3, 'Relating', therefore discusses the feeling body from the perspectives of biology, social science and psychology, and it shows that from within all three fields the body is open to relational and cultural influence. It is argued that, despite the many differences between them, with respect to the feeling body both social science and psychology converge upon the issues raised by notions of determinism, consciousness and agency.

Some implications of the discussions set out in the previous two chapters are elaborated with respect to notions of experience in Chapter 4, 'Experiencing'. Focusing on the interplay of feeling and language, the chapter explores the origins and character of feelings of knowing and discusses the role of habit in stabilising experience and constituting subjectivities. Drawing on various resources including Vygotsky and Shotter as well as Langer, experience is characterised as a felt-discursive 'boundary phenomenon', always being remade in the flux of social relations.

Since an emphasis on feeling has various implications for methodology, Chapter 5, 'Researching', considers a series of issues raised, or likely to be encountered, by empirical analyses of feeling. The implications of these issues for both quantitative and qualitative research are considered, and some potential methodological strategies for addressing them are briefly outlined. After this, the emphasis of the book shifts and the next three chapters present more empirically oriented analyses that demonstrate how our psychological understanding of particular topics is changed by an analysis that explicitly incorporates feeling.

In Chapter 6, 'Believing', psychological notions of belief are discussed in relation to matters of health and illness. A definition of belief as an organisation of feeling contingently allied to discourse is described and explained. The example of religiosity/spirituality and its relationship to health and illness is then used to demonstrate how this conception of belief may shed additional light upon research findings. The chapter also discusses health beliefs as they appear within social cognition models of health behaviour and as they are associated with tobacco-smoking.

Towards the end of this chapter, it is suggested that 'sensibility' might be a better term to use in relation to those relatively diverse organisations of discourse and feeling that are more typically called health beliefs. Chapter 7, 'Exhausting', therefore analyses some data that suggest how feeling, knowledge and corporeal practice could come together for some people given the diagnosis of chronic fatigue syndrome (CFS). The analysis proposes that a particular sensibility might be acquired by some people with this diagnosis, as a joint consequence both of their efforts to manage its symptoms and to take heed of relevant medical advice. At the same time, medical professionals may develop their own contrasting sensibility with respect to their practice, and the discordances between this and the modal sensibility identified in relation to CFS might account for some of the negative stereotypes associated with this diagnosis.

Since both beliefs and sensibilities are associated with mental health and illness, Chapter 8, 'Maddening', discusses how clinical paranoia and madness – associated with the psychiatric diagnosis of schizophrenia and with notions of psychosis – might be constituted from complex mixtures of enduring feeling locked into place by social, relational and material circumstances. Whilst many feelings are relevant to these states, fear, shame and anger may be especially prominent. The concept of 'feeling traps' is introduced and, in conjunction with the phenomena of habituation to emotional feelings, used to explain the relational constitution of so-called 'florid' states.

Finally, Chapter 9, 'Concluding', draws the book to a close by briefly situating feeling with respect to two relevant bodies of work. First, feeling is discussed in relation to scholarship in the social sciences and humanities associated with the affective turn. Two examples – the use of music during forcible interrogation, and the culture of fear that is said to inhabit contemporary politics – are used to ground a discussion comparing notions of affect with notions of feeling. These examples also begin to illustrate some of the wider relevance of the concepts discussed in this book. Finally, some issues that a psychology of feeling might encounter are identified and the dangers and potentials associated with them are briefly assessed.

# 2
# Feeling

In a shifting myriad of ways, feelings are intrinsically part of experience. This chapter will detail what feelings are, describe how they are the most fundamental constituents of experience and discuss ways of categorising or classifying them for analytic purposes. The arguments are informed by the writings of Maurice Merleau-Ponty, John Shotter, William Stern and Mark Johnson, along with other scholarship associated with the affective turn. However, the primary influence is the three volumes of Susanne Langer's work *Mind: An Essay on Human Feeling*.

## A process philosophy of feeling

Susanne Langer was born in 1895 in New York and died in 1985. Her parents were German immigrants to the USA (her father was a partner in a bank), so she grew up speaking English and German, then learned French at school. She displayed a precocious talent for philosophy and is said to have read Kant's *Critique of Pure Reason* before she was 12 years old. Langer had an abiding interest in art and was a synaesthete who perceived specific colours in relation to particular vowel sounds (Langer, 1967, p. 195).

Langer's doctoral studies were supervised by Alfred North Whitehead, whose influence permeates her work. Her bestselling book *Philosophy in a New Key*, published in 1941, was also influenced by her reading of Cassirer (including her translation into English of his *Language and Myth*). Cassirer's analyses of culture and poetry helped Langer extend her early interest in logic and symbolism beyond the formal symbols of language and mathematics, to develop a philosophy of art. Her trilogy *Mind: An Essay on Human Feeling* (Langer, 1967, 1972, 1982) is in many ways a development of these earlier interests. In *Mind* she is frequently concerned with symbolism; she explicitly recognises some of the limits of language (in a fashion informed by the early Wittgenstein); and she displays a constant interest in feeling, sensation and perception and their intimate, constitutive connections with reasoning and being. Her aim in this work seems to be the development of "a kind of semiotic psychology that is not cut off from its biological roots" (Innis, 2009, p. 153).

The most obvious way in which Whitehead's influence over Langer is evident is that, like his, hers is a process philosophy. In *Mind*, Langer tries to explicate how the world comes to be for us as a consequence of ongoing processes within our bodies and of prior (evolutionary) processes that have endowed our bodies with particular capacities and sensibilities. Whether discussing phenomenological experiences, biological processes or evolutionary changes, Langer constantly emphasises rhythms, flows, feedback and feed-forward loops, circuits, entrainments and other temporally organised movements of becoming and actualisation.[1] Consequently, she frequently undercuts taken-for-granted dualisms – between nature and nurture, mind and body, and biology and culture. Langer's analyses demonstrate how, when examined over time, such supposedly separate entities actually infuse, shape and mutually constitute each other.

However, Langer also diverges from Whitehead, largely because his aim was metaphysics whilst hers was a philosophy of mind.[2] This difference is reflected in their conceptualisations of the term 'experience'. Whitehead is sometimes described as a pan-experientialist, because he uses 'experience' to describe every kind of process or activity between every kind of entity – including, for example, activities solely involving atoms and molecules. He conceptualises experience as a general capacity to respond that does not require awareness and, indeed, is often conducted by entities constitutionally incapable of reflexive consciousness.[3] Consistent with her aim to produce a philosophy of mind, however, Langer conceives of 'experience' solely in relation to biological capacities. She does not differentiate sharply between human experience and that of other animals, nor does she see an absolute distinction between experience now and experience in the distant (evolutionary) past: she simply reserves the term 'experience' solely for living creatures.

As the subtitle of *Mind* signals, Langer treats feeling as the primordial raw material of experience: before anything else, experience consists of feeling. Feeling, however, is not a substance or thing: it is a mobile, fluctuating, emergent phase of organic life. Although we sometimes talk freely of 'having a feeling', this is a category error because "Feeling is a verbal noun – a noun made out of a verb, that psychologically makes an entity out of a process. To feel is to do something, not to have something" (Langer, 1967, p. 20). In other words, feeling falls into the category of activities and processes, not the category of things and substances: "the phenomena usually described as 'a feeling' is really that an organism feels something, i.e. that something is felt. What is felt is a process, perhaps a large complex of processes, within the organism" (Langer, 1967, p. 21).

In this way, Langer begins breaking down the presumed separation between feeling, as an aspect of experience or phenomenology, and the body as a material, biological entity. It is not that there is a body to which an additional property, feeling, sometimes gets added. There is simply a living body which is continuously active, even when this activity consists solely of maintaining itself by monitoring, regulating and balancing its many processes. The body, here, includes the brain, since it is by cultural convention rather than anatomical necessity that we place the boundary of the brain somewhere near the base of the skull. Physically, the brain permeates the entire body, its spinal cord and peripheral nerves radiating from head to fingers to toes. Simultaneously, the entire nervous system, including those parts within the skull, is constantly awash with changing levels of different molecules – hormones, peptides, neurotransmitters, enzymes and so on. Damasio (1994) neatly summarises the inseparability of body and brain when he says that not only is the brain embodied, the body is also 'embrained'.

So the living body – which includes the brain – is always enacting multiple processes, typically in concert, such that in effect the body is a self-assembling locus of activity. When this activity crosses a threshold of intensity, the body enters the phase we call feeling. Langer explains this using the analogy of an iron bar in a flame: "When iron is heated to a critical degree it becomes red; yet its redness is not a new entity which must have gone somewhere else when it is no longer in the iron. It was a phase of the iron itself, at high temperature" (Langer, 1967, p. 21). So feeling emerges as a quality or aspect of the body under certain conditions, when it adopts a particular orientation, or is charged by a specific impetus – just as redness emerges when iron becomes sufficiently hot.

Langer was writing before contemporary neuroscience enabled more specificity about the many brain regions that seem important for enabling different kinds of feeling. These regions are *not* 'the parts of the brain that produce feeling' – they are simply structures and regions frequently implicated in the particular kinds of felt experience that have thus far been studied (predominantly, emotional experiences and pain).

Amongst others, these regions include the amygdala, hypothalamus, cingulate gyrus, insula, the parietal lobe, parts of the brainstem and areas of the ventro-medial prefrontal cortex. The identification of these regions updates Langer's claim by lending it a little more putative specificity. At the same time, these brain areas only enable feeling within complex, variable, distributed neural networks, and in conjunction with multiple body-brain systems.[4] Their identification is therefore compatible with Langer's claim that the body's many interlocking, mutually regulating processes (neural, vascular, hormonal, physiological, autonomic, sensory, gustatory, kinaesthetic and more) place it constantly in flux and that combinations of processes may cross a threshold, beyond which the body enters the phase of being felt.

Langer notes that this threshold is somewhat mobile, a product of other processes and of fluctuating environmental impingements. A hand plunged into lukewarm water might feel intense heat if first immersed in ice. Anger might be felt more readily, or with greater force, if preceded by anxiety; conversely, it might be felt in a more attenuated fashion if preceding circumstances are suffused with feelings of affection. Again, aspects of contemporary neuroscience illuminate and perhaps extend Langer's claim. Damasio (1999) proposes that feeling consists not so much of increased intensities as of changes from one bodily state to another: that feeling consists of the *difference* between the current state of the body-brain system and that immediately preceding. Difference, here, includes changes in the character of feeling, as well as changes in intensity.[5] But whether feeling is conceived solely as the product of intensity, or whether it can also be conceived as the product of difference, it is always generated by multiple body–brain systems. These systems monitor, regulate and dynamically maintain the body's integrity and preparedness, allowing us to act in, and react to, changing social, relational, environmental and material circumstances.

Understood as a continuous potential of the living body, feeling is much more than a component of emotion. Feeling is a much broader and fundamental capacity, the very stuff of experience itself. Whilst emotions typically contain prominent felt elements – the sweaty palms of fear, the burning face of shame, the clenched gut of anger – feeling is a universal capacity within experience more generally. Langer argues that feeling is the source, the beginning, the constitutive material from which and upon which all of our more usual psychological categories are differentiated: "the entire psychological field – including human conception, responsible action, rationality, knowledge – is a vast and branching development of feeling" (Langer, 1967, p. 22). This startling claim, which *Mind* sets out to demonstrate, has three far-reaching implications.

First, this claim signals that feeling is profoundly *constitutive* of experience, rather than being simply something that, sometimes, appears within it. Langer proposes that *all* of the processes that make up experience – 'the entire psychological field' – can be traced back, in part, to feeling. Feeling is already part of what we call conceptualisation, decision-making, judgement and rationality. What we call conceptualisation, for example, begins with feeling, as does what we call decision-making (responsible action, in Langer's terms). However, this does not mean that conceiving and deciding are somehow irrational, because feeling is also part of rationality.

In our culture and psychology, we are used to equating feeling and emotion with irrationality and excess, treating them as the polar opposites of rational judgement and consideration. As Langer puts it:

> Reason and feeling, logic and emotion, intellect and passion or however we name the incompatible pair, are most commonly treated as two opposed principles of motivation which can be reconciled only by striking a balance between them, sacrificing much passion, sympathy and gratification of desire to reason, and a little rational judgement to the admitted 'natural affections'.
>
> (Langer, 1967, p. 148)

Psychological notions of mental ill health, for example, often associate excesses of emotion and feeling with irrational thoughts and actions. Similarly, when psychology models processes of deciding, judging or evaluating it does so predominantly in terms of information flows and cognitive variables, producing flow diagrams within which feelings – if included at all – commonly play a subsidiary or interfering role. Feelings, emotions or affects are typically positioned either as irrelevant to effective reasoning and rational decision-making or as obstacles to them:

> Most cognitive psychologists conducting research have chosen to ignore the issue of the effects of emotions on cognition by attempting to keep the emotional state of their subjects constant... As there are almost constant interactions between cognition and emotion in everyday life, any attempt to provide an adequate theory of cognition that ignores emotion is probably doomed to failure.
>
> (Eysenck, 1991, p. 435, in Wilson, 1999)

Dixon (2003) shows how the notion that feeling necessarily impedes rationality is historically specific. He demonstrates that during the 18th and 19th centuries an entire palette of affective concepts – including appetites, sentiments, affections and passions – was gradually replaced by a single over-arching category of emotion. This shift was associated with the decline of Christian influence, the increased secularisation of European and American thought and the rise of science. It eventually produced the more mechanical, automatic, modern concept of emotion, and it was the emergence of this modern concept that created its relatively sharp separation from concepts of rationality and intellect. Previously, Dixon suggests, more nuanced and subtle discussions of the relations between thinking and feeling could be had. Dixon's claims echo recent work in neuroscience which not only suggests that feeling and emotion contribute to rational deliberation and decision-making but also finds that deficits in feeling (as a consequence of neurological impairment) are frequently associated with impaired decision-making and poor judgement (e.g. Bechara, Damasio, Damasio, & Lee, 1999).

Langer's claim regarding the intrinsic contribution of feeling to rationality is also compatible with the observation that there are different rationalities, each with associated orchestrations of feeling. This can be understood by starting from the societal level: for example, under the ideology of Nazism in Germany it was considered rational to execute adults and children with disabilities, who were described as *lebensunwertes leben* or 'life unworthy of life'. This rationality was an element of the eugenic thinking which was influential (and associated with progressive politics) in the USA, the UK and Sweden, as well as Germany (Macey, 2009). Under the Nazis, however, eugenics shaped medical discourses and informed medical school training in particular ways. Doctors were instructed to re-conceptualise health as the health of the 'race' rather than the individual, and so encouraged to overcome their feelings of shame and revulsion at deliberately killing vulnerable people (Lifton, 1986).

Simultaneously, the notion that there are different rationalities with associated orchestrations of feeling can be understood by starting from individual experience. Willig (1995) investigated why people in established relationships often quickly stop using condoms, even though neither they nor their partners may have been tested for sexually transmitted diseases. Her participants described condom use as signalling feelings of mistrust, and abandoning condoms as part of cementing relationships and sharing new levels of intimacy. Not using condoms becomes entirely 'rational' when the powerful needs and feelings of a new relationship trump the muted feelings of anxiety associated with the abstract risk of contracting an STD.

Jaggar (1989) argues that dominant notions of rationality are already predicated upon a particular, gendered organisation of knowledge with respect to feeling. The positivist view that rationality is achieved by excluding emotion in fact reflects the ways of embodied being commonly exhibited in American and European cultures by white men:

> Modern Western men, in contrast with Shakespeare's heroes, for instance, are required to present a facade of coolness, lack of excitement, even boredom, to express emotion only rarely and then for relatively trivial events, such as sporting occasions, where the emotions expressed are acknowledged to be dramatized and so are not taken entirely seriously. Thus, women in our society form the main group allowed or even expected to express emotion. A woman may cry in the face of disaster, and a man of color may gesticulate, but a white man merely sets his jaw.
>
> (Jaggar, 1989, p. 164)

Our dominant notion of rationality is associated with a particular, corresponding organisation of feeling wherein emotion is denied, suppressed or controlled, and its uninhibited expression is associated with subordinate or marginalised groups. The view that rational reasoning and accurate knowledge are necessarily dispassionate and cool therefore reinforces existing social hierarchies because it functions

> to bolster the epistemic authority of the currently dominant groups, composed largely of white men, and to discredit the observations and claims of the currently subordinate groups including, of course, the observations and claims of many people of color and women. The more forcefully and vehemently the latter groups express their observations and claims, the more emotional they appear and so the more easily they are discredited. The alleged epistemic authority of the dominant groups then justifies their political authority.
>
> (Jaggar, 1989, pp. 164–165)

These three examples begin to show how rationalities, *as they get lived*, are not only cultural and historical but also situated and local. Everyday rationalities instantiate, rather than transcend, normative compulsions and individual interests, and in each case their instantiation is bound up with a particular, corresponding orchestration of feeling. Feeling is the basic raw material from which other psychological capacities, including the ability to reason, get differentiated, so that "the wide discrepancy between reason and feeling may be unreal; it is not improbable that intellect is a high form of feeling – a specialised, intensive feeling about intuitions" (Langer, 1967, p. 149).

Langer's claim further implies that feeling is constitutive in the sense that it is, primordially, what experience is made from. It is not so much that we *have* feelings, because this way of talking misrepresents a phase of activity as a thing or substance. It is more that *feelings have us*: the process of feeling makes us – or, at least, makes our experience. Feeling constitutes experience *before* logical reflection and is, in fact, the primary process from which all reflection proceeds. So we can't simply turn around on our feelings to objectively interrogate them, because our 'turning around' is already shaped by the feelings we wish to interpret. This is one reason we cannot necessarily give accurate self-reports of our own psychological processes, although there are others (e.g. Kahneman, 2012).

Second, Langer's claim that "the entire psychological field...is a vast and branching development of feeling" is a decisive rejection of the Cartesian (mind–body) dualism which is largely taken for granted in our culture, and which (as Chapter 1 argued) is firmly entrenched within psychology. There are two main senses in which we can understand Cartesian dualism in psychology, and Langer's claim challenges both. In the first sense, we have minds and we have bodies and these are separate entities forged of different substances. In the second sense, we are Cartesian subjects, the disembodied occupants of a 'Cartesian theatre' from within which we dispassionately view the world.

Langer's claim challenges Cartesian dualism in this first sense because it implies that all the things we think of as our minds are aspects of the processes of our bodies. It is not that these psychological capacities do not exist, nor that they can be dismissed as mere epiphenomena, and certainly not that they can be reduced to bodily processes. It is simply that they cannot be separated from the bodies of which they are emergent properties – first as feelings, and subsequently as the many psychological categories into which feeling differentiates. Mind is constituted of feeling, and feeling is a phase or aspect of the body: these are not separable elements made of different substances.

Instead of accepting 'mind' as a metaphysically ultimate reality, distinct from the physical reality which subsumes the brain, and asking how the two can 'make liaison', one may hope to describe 'mind' as a phenomenon in terms of the highest physiological processes, especially those which have psychical phases.

(Langer, 1967, p. 29)

Langer's claim also challenges Cartesian dualism insofar as it implies that we are transcendent subjects dispassionately observing the world. Feelings constitute experience, which means that they also, simultaneously and mutually, constitute us as experiencing subjects. Suppose, I find myself outside a cake shop whilst hungry. My feelings of hunger constitute the cakes as having significance and value, endowing them with a kind of magnetic pull, whilst simultaneously constituting me as someone for whom cakes are relevant and good. I am not a transcendent Cartesian subject, dispassionately observing cakes as objects. I am an *immanent* subject (Brown & Stenner, 2009) with a pre-reflective, felt, interest-laden relation with cakes. Although it can be more difficult to appreciate this immanent relationship when objects less 'interesting' than cakes are involved, Langer proposes that it often becomes visible in dreams, which are frequently structured by movements, arcs and eruptions of feeling.

Third, Langer's claim challenges the relatively sharp distinction that psychology typically makes between cognition and affect, or thought and emotion; moreover, it does so in a particularly interesting way. In asserting that 'the entire psychological field' branches or differentiates from feeling, Langer first rejects the idea that the categories of cognition and affect are separate and distinct – a controversial move for those who treat cognition as the dominant element of human psychology. Cognitive psychology is organised around notions of information processing derived from cybernetics, information theory, computer simulation, artificial intelligence and mathematical modelling (Gardner, 1985) where cognition is presumed to be (at least in principle) separate from affect and not dependent upon dynamics of feeling.

It has previously been noted, however, that psychology embraces many constructs which, although superficially (treated as) cognitive, are consistently associated with, penetrated by or shot through with feeling. High self-esteem is associated with feelings of confidence, being valued and having influence or power. Self-efficacy is associated with feelings of competence, mastery and ability. Attitudes are typically conceptualised as cognitive (although they are more accurately discursive) but are nevertheless frequently enacted through feelings towards their object. Even highly skilled expertise, based upon accumulated knowledge and ready familiarity with rules and principles, is associated with a 'feel for' the task at hand. Such considerations lead Wilson (1999, p. 142) to argue that, despite superficial impressions, cognitive psychology has not actually ignored emotion: instead, "mainstream cognitivism has *marginalised* affect...it has split cognition from the affects and pursued cognition without considering the influence of the affects".

In some quarters, the psychological divide between cognition and affect is now being questioned. Phelps (2006) summarises research into the functions of the amygdala, identifying five areas of research that demonstrate the interaction of emotion and cognition, and to which amygdala function is relevant: emotional learning; emotion and memory; emotion, attention and perception; emotion and social stimuli processing; and changing emotional responses through emotion regulation. In each area, Phelps finds evidence that "the division of human behaviour into emotion and cognition is not as clear as previous philosophical and psychological investigations have suggested" (Phelps, 2006, p. 46). For example, there is evidence that where attentional resources are limited, emotionally laden stimuli are more likely to reach awareness than neutral ones, demonstrating that emotion can shape subsequent cognition. Conversely, there is also evidence that contextual information presented in language can modulate amygdala fear responses, suggesting that language processing can shape affective reactions.

Similar questioning is occurring in neuroscience. Whilst there are relatively distinct fields of cognitive and affective neuroscience, some scholars increasingly understand these distinctions as flags of convenience, ways of defining a set of topical priorities rather than strategies for carving nature at its joints. Summarising some of the relevant evidence, Duncan and Barrett (2007, pp. 1187–1188) say:

> [P]arts of the brain that have traditionally been called 'cognitive' participate in instantiating an affective state, not merely regulating that state after it has been established. Furthermore, the parts of the brain that have traditionally been called 'affective' participate in cognitive processes. The so-called 'affective' brain areas (e.g., the amygdala and brainstem) participate in sensory processing and contribute to consciousness in a manner that meets most definitions of 'cognition'.

Chapter 1 described how the two most influential current theories in emotion science – Scherer's component process model, and Feldman-Barrett's core affect theory – both conceptualise emotions as consisting of cognitive *and* affective elements. Moreover, even scholars who argue for distinct cognitive and affective systems nevertheless acknowledge that causality between them is bi-directional and that "emotions and cognitions are continually interacting in almost all mental activities" (Ciompi & Panksepp, 2005, p. 23). Unsurprisingly, then, the view that cognition and affect are not separate is now gaining ground in contemporary psychological research.

However, Langer is not only suggesting that cognition and affect are inseparable. She also proposes that feeling comes first – that the processes we call thought are just as much a development of feeling as those we call emotion. Langer does not treat these different facets of experience as homogenous or uniform: she simply proposes that (what we call) cognition, or thought, and (what we call) affect, or emotion, are elaborated branches of a single fundamental process – feeling. The process of feeling is a capacity of organic creatures, the continuous potential to generate a living psychology grounded in, though not determined by, the organismic processes of being:

> Feeling is the constant, systematic, but private display of what is going on in our own system, the index of much that goes on below the limen of sentience, and ultimately of the whole organic process, or life, that feeds and uses the sensory and cerebral system.
>
> (Langer, 1967, p. 58)

If it's challenging disciplinary aspects are temporarily set aside, Langer's claim might be questioned on experiential grounds. When we reflect upon our experience, feeling might not seem to be constantly present, and it may not obviously contribute to all of our psychological processes. So if feeling is part of every experience, the root of all psychological capacities, why is this not obvious? A discussion of analytic categories of feeling, and of its various qualities, will enable a return to this question at the end of this chapter.

### Analytic categories of feeling

Langer (1967, p. 23) suggests that "[t]he most important distinction within the realm of feeling is between what is felt as impact and what is felt as autogenic action"; that is, between feelings associated with external events or stimulations and those associated with internal ones. Langer relates this categorisation to the distinction, dominant in the psychology of her time, between stimulus and response, and it has a consistent significance in her account of the development of mind and symbolisation. However, she acknowledges considerable complexity in relation to this seemingly simple distinction. Consonant with her rejection of the Cartesian divide between subject and object, she proposes that "by 'subjective' I mean whatever is felt as action, and by 'objective' whatever is felt as impact" (Langer, 1967, p. 31). In other words, the distinction is effectively an experiential one, based upon what is *felt as* originating either internally or externally. In actuality, because the body is always in the world, the feelings it enables always reflect world and body simultaneously – albeit that we then typically categorise them as either primarily internal or primarily external.

Whilst Langer's distinction is important, it leaves considerable detail unresolved. Addressing this, I have proposed (Cromby, 2007) that feelings can be seen as falling into three fuzzy-edged analytic categories. The first category contains *emotional feelings*. Whilst emotions are complex phenomena combining cultural, historical, cognitive, felt, motivational and enactive components, they all include a notable embodied element: the sinking feeling of dread, the hot face of anger, the dead weight of sadness, the 'butterflies in the stomach' of anxiety and so on. If these bodily elements could somehow be extracted from the complexes to which they are integral, these are what would be referred to as emotional feelings.[6]

The second category can be called *extra-emotional feelings*. Some of these feelings are associated with bodily needs and impulses – for example, pain, hunger, tiredness, alertness, sexual desire. Other feelings in this category are more overtly relational, associated with being comforted, tickled, massaged, stroked, caressed, pushed, held and so on. This terminology acknowledges that these feelings typically have emotional elements bound up with them. The emotional dimensions of hunger and satiation are frequently prominent in the lives of people given psychiatric diagnoses of eating disorders (Meyer, Waller, & Waters, 1998). Pain has an affective component (e.g. Rhudy et al., 2006), and sexual desire is freighted with multiple, and sometimes conflicting, emotional meanings (Hiller, 2005). Likewise, depending on its emotional and relational context, tickling can be either pleasant or painful (Phillips, 1994), just as stroking, touching and holding in general can be intrusive, disturbing, claustrophobic, reassuring, relaxing or energising, according to the social and relational situations within which they occur.

So to describe these feelings as extra-emotional is not to deny their emotional aspects, rather to emphasise that emotion does not exhaustively eliminate them. If the emotions could be stripped away, meaningful residues would remain that reflected the needs or stimulations that prompted them. Severe pain, for example, has distinct phenomenological qualities that differentiate it from other unpleasant feelings (Scarry, 1985; Leder, 1990). Likewise, although psychology frequently characterises them both as appetites or motivations, hunger does not feel the same as sexual desire: each has what can be called a different *texture*.

The third category is *feelings of knowing*. This category encompasses the many, subtle, fleeting feelings that arise in relationships and social interactions, as well as in deliberation, reasoning and decision-making. They are the feelings associated with half-formed desires, inarticulate refusals, the imperfect sense of a significance not yet fully realised, a decision tentatively made, a judgement only partially realised or an understanding not wholly articulated. They are feelings for which, in English at least, we have few words, although the umbrella term 'gut feelings' is sometimes used. William James discussed these feelings in relation to intellectual tasks, associating them with the words we use to signal acts of reasoning, judgement and evaluation: "We ought to say a feeling of and, a feeling of if, a feeling of but, and a feeling of by, quite as readily as we say a feeling of blue or a feeling of cold" (James, 1892). Johnson (2007) relates these intellectual feelings to his work with Lakoff on metaphors, proposing that they are primarily enabled by the sensori-motor cortex and that they play a vital role in guiding reasoning and thinking.

Simultaneously, these feelings play a vital part in our relationships. Shotter (1993a, 1993b) calls them "knowing of the third kind", describing them as an indispensable part of "joint action": the way in which spontaneous social interactions unfurl in a mutually responsive manner, where the utterances of each person are tailored into a co-created evolving context of background expectations. As we talk with another, we continuously register their posture, gestures and facial expressions, the cadences, rhythms and intonations of their speech, its emphases, pauses and gaps. This creates for us a felt sense of how the interaction is proceeding, allowing us to *feel* how we might next respond.

Although these three analytic categories reflect phenomenological and functional differences, our everyday experience of feeling is frequently more fluid and indecipherable. One issue is that emotional feelings can also be conceptual: my flash of anger at an unreasonable work demand is part of my growing realisation that my job is becoming intolerable. Additionally, since feeling is the emergent consequence of multiple simultaneous processes, it is always moving and changing. Consequently, feelings are sometimes mixed, vacillating or confused (e.g. Sullivan & Strongman, 2003), their multiple flows reflecting changing bodily needs, situations and environments, shifting relational imperatives, and often contradictory social positions. Moreover, as scholars of affect have emphasised, feelings are typically responsive to those of significant others. Sometimes they are attuned, such that our feelings resonate with theirs, and this we call empathy; at other times, how we feel is responsive in a discordant manner. A lover's need for reassurance might elicit sympathy and concern; alternately, it might produce impatience. In each case, our feelings are responsive, and in each case readily give rise to further feelings. I, or my lover, might take my impatience as an object and then be sad, angry or confused because of it; I in turn might feel ashamed, anxious or tired by this reaction. Complex intra- and interpersonal circuits of feeling can ensue, where mutually interpellated multiple feeling states are enacted, sometimes in rapid succession.

It has already been noted that we do not always know why we feel as we do. Feelings can be elicited by transient features of environments, situations or relations that, whilst registered, do not necessarily become the focus of reflection and awareness. Hence, subtle feelings of familiarity render consumers more readily prey to advertisers' efforts to inculcate brand loyalty (Ha & Perks, 2005), whilst feelings of mastery, domination, exclusion and difference are continuously yet almost imperceptibly interpellated by mainstream cultural presentations of marginalised groups (Grossberg, 1992). Moreover, we often have good reasons to pretend that we – or others – are not experiencing particular feelings. These disavowals may function to avoid hurting or embarrassing a loved one, to endure a situation that might otherwise be unbearable, or protect against understandings that – at least for now – are too difficult to accept.

### Descriptive qualities of feeling

Alongside these analytic categories, it is necessary to have an agreed language with which to talk about feeling. This is difficult, since it involves using words to indicate qualities of experience that are fundamentally not linguistic: ultimately, this means there is something inescapably metaphorical about any language used to describe feelings. Nevertheless, we can and do talk about feelings, and any systematic analysis demands an appropriate terminology: with this in mind, Table 2.1 provides some useful terms.

The column of general qualities is informed by discussions of emotion and of bodily sensations such as pain,[7] and contains coarse dimensions along which most feelings can be arrayed. The terms are largely

*Table 2.1*   A terminology for qualities of feeling

| General qualities | Meaning qualities | Temporal qualities |
| --- | --- | --- |
| Intensity | Association | Crescendo |
| Valence | Obstruction | Decrescendo |
| Location | Connection | Bursting |
| Duration | Disjunction | Surging |
| Texture | Contradiction | Fading |
| | Rightness | Fleeting |
| | Completion | Drawn-out |
| | | Explosive |

self-explanatory, with the exception of texture: as noted earlier, texture refers to how feelings that might be functionally related are nevertheless experientially different: for example, how hunger differs from sexual desire. The column of meaning qualities is largely drawn from Johnson (2007), although some terms from Langer are also included. Whilst it refers most obviously to feelings of knowing, such qualities may also be related to extra-emotional or emotional feelings: touching and being touched can create feelings of connection, just as feelings of connection might arise as nuances of feelings of love or affection. The column of temporal qualities, finally, offers terms that describe how feelings are orchestrated across time. They come from Stern (1985) who deployed them in a study of mother–child interaction. He described these aspects of feeling as 'vitality affects' which are "inextricably involved with all the vital processes of life, such as breathing, getting hungry, eliminating, falling asleep and emerging out of sleep, or feeling the comings and goings of emotions and thoughts" (op. cit., p. 54). Stern's terminology adds useful nuance to Langer's characterisation of arcs of feeling in terms of gradients and rhythms.

So feelings can be categorised as arising primarily from external forces or impacts, or from internal events or autogenic processes. They can also be categorised as emotional or extra-emotional, and as feelings of knowing. Cutting across these categories, feelings have qualities such as location, intensity, valence, duration and texture. But they also have other important features, associated with their rates of velocity and acceleration and with their a-representational and immediate status.

## Feelings: Velocity and acceleration

Feelings are the product of process, and process extends over time: consequently, the temporal qualities of feeling are always potentially relevant. Connolly's (2002) analyses of feeling and time show how feelings are sometimes slower to come, and slower to depart, than other aspects of experience. A brief distressing interaction might leave a growing feeling of sadness, and this feeling might develop and linger for hours. Conversely, the feeling of profound insight when we recognise in an instant that something is wrong – or indeed right – can arise very suddenly, such that our discursive reasoning then struggles to catch up with and articulate our felt understanding.

Because feelings can move at different speeds and accelerate at different rates to other aspects of experience, they have the continuous potential to be out of phase with them. Although feelings frequently align themselves with present concerns, at other times they are discordant, and these discordances themselves have temporal qualities – they may, for example, be growing or surging, or they may be drawn out and diminishing. It is this potential for feelings to be out of phase with other elements of experience that supplies their occasional disruptive force, just as their potential to synchronise with other elements enables them to reinforce accepted practices and understandings. Feelings can reproduce and maintain existing patterns of relating and being, and they can also disrupt and subvert them: they are not necessarily agents of change, but nor are they necessarily elements of the status quo.

### Feelings: Immediate and a-representational

Feelings are embodied, and bodily experience is ineffable: this is why films, visual images, dance, emoticons and music – channels of communication not wholly dependent upon language and symbols – are so effective at communicating feeling. It is also why, when we use language to communicate feeling, we regularly employ similes and metaphors: my anger was burning; I was dragged down by the weight of tiredness; I felt so confused my head was spinning. Each of these short phrases attempts to convey in words something felt with the body. Whilst each suggests something of the feelings they are meant to relay, each falls short of precisely representing them. We think we know what they mean, but it is always possible we are wrong: perhaps your burning anger does not actually feel anything like mine?

In other words, feelings are *a-representational*. Although frequently highly significant, their significance is not primarily because of anything they represent or stand for. If someone we love dies suddenly, we might feel shock, anxiety and sadness. But it will make little sense to treat these feelings as standing for, or representing, something about this death: rather, they actually constitute many of its significances. Suppose instead that our loved one had a long, fulfilling life, but had been in intense pain with an incurable condition: our sadness might then be tinged with bitter-sweet feelings of relief. Conversely, news of the death of someone whose life and work never impacted upon us in any noticeable way is unlikely to arouse any intense feelings (unless their death is an iconic event capable of luring feelings associated with our own circumstances – Brown, Basil, & Bocarnea, 2003).

None of this is to say that feelings associated with bereavement are meaningless, but to observe that their meaning is not a function of anything they represent: it is a function of what they *do*, the potentials they realise and the changes they instantiate. Instead of representing the relationship we previously had with our loved one, feelings of shock, grief and sadness are lived elements within its profound transformation by their death. Their meanings arise in and of the lived moments of our bereavement and are fully sensible only as components within it (Cromby & Phillips, 2014).

Feelings are not only a-representational, they also have the quality of immediacy: we experience our feelings *immediately*, sensuously, through the lived flesh. 'Immediate', here, has two meanings. First, feelings arise spontaneously, pre-reflectively and without bidding. They are notoriously resistant to willed effort: if not there would be little need for clinical psychology, notions of 'will power' would never have emerged, and skilled theatrical performers would not be praised. Second, feelings arise before the conventionalised reflections they (almost instantaneously) co-constitute: rather than being initially mediated by these reflections, they are im-mediate.[8]

These qualities of a-representationality and immediacy help explain how, whilst feeling sometimes captures attention, it often remains in the background. It is not uncommon to encounter people who appear to imagine themselves calm and relaxed, yet whose very being throbs with concern. Similarly we may sometimes notice how the words of call-centre workers seem saturated by a complex of felt tensions, presumably reflective of the incentives and penalties within which they are enmeshed, and how these tensions – more than the scripts they follow – impel their telephone manner. Or we might not realise that we feel anxious until someone points out that we seem unable to sit still; might find ourselves feeling impatient, and gradually become aware that we feel hungry: or might strive to ignore feelings of resentment at an inequitable situation, only to wonder why we subsequently feel listless and numb.

Paradoxical as it might sound, then, feelings can be influential merely as organic states of the body-brain system, as well as phenomenological experiences of those states: feelings do not have to be attended to, reflected upon or noticed in order to have some influence.[9] To an extent this is because – despite its continuous presence – feeling is often not the focus of our attention. In Langer's words:

> The real patterns of feeling – how a small fright, or 'startle', terminates; how the tensions of boredom increase or give way to self-entertainment, how daydreaming weaves in and out of realistic thought, how the feeling of a place, a time of day, an ordinary situation is built up – these felt events, which compose the fabric of mental life, usually pass unobserved, unrecorded and therefore essentially unknown to the average person.
>
> (Langer, 1967, p. 57)

One reason feeling tends to fall into the background is that it is frequently more adaptive to engage with the person, activity or phenomena prompting it. But this adaptive tendency combines with the intrinsic qualities of feeling: its variable speeds and rates of acceleration, its immediacy and a-representational character, its ineffability. Together, this generates propensities to primarily recall only the discursive-symbolic-representational elements that we used to represent, communicate and organise our experience, the prominence of which means we often ignore, fail to notice and therefore quickly forget the fluid-immediate-ineffable flows of feeling that prompted them, motivated their selection, guided their evaluation, organised their relevances, and constituted the judgements we made of them. In this way, despite their continual influence, many feelings come and go without our properly noticing them.

We can now return to the question posed earlier: if feelings are part of *all* of our experiences, why is this not more obvious? First, we are misled by cultural and psychological tendencies to presume that reasoning and deciding are not already bound up with feeling, and to solely equate feeling with relatively distinct emotional episodes. Second, feelings are embodied, so necessarily ineffable, immediate and a-representational. Third, they are always moving and changing, sometimes at speeds and rates that exceed or elude reflection. Fourth, many feelings are fleeting, subtle, somewhat amorphous, hard to locate corporeally, and not readily concordant with any widely used terminology. And fifth, whilst their influence is continuous it operates before representation and precedes formal conceptualisation. As Langer (1967, p. 57) puts it:

> It may seem strange that the most immediate experiences in our lives should be the least recognised, but there is a reason for this apparent paradox, and the reason is precisely their immediacy. They pass unrecorded because they are known without any symbolic mediation, and therefore without conceptual form.

## Feeling body, social world

So Langer proposes that feelings are not just emotions, nor even just aspects of emotions. They are emergent phases of the body that continuously suffuse awareness and co-constitute all experience – the 'entire psychological field'. But unless they are especially acute, sudden or prolonged, feelings nevertheless tend to drop into the background, leading us to underestimate their contribution.

Despite its strengths, Langer's account is incomplete because, whilst social influence is discussed, it is not always considered in sufficient detail. Shotter's (1993a) analysis of deciding when to first say 'I love you' in a new relationship illustrates what is largely missing. He shows how feeling vitally informs this decision, which is necessarily a momentous one because – however the declaration is received – the relationship will be irreversibly transformed. Here, as in every other instance of relating, what I feel is continuously responsive to (my sense of) what you feel – just as your feelings are simultaneously and continuously responsive to (your sense of) mine. But Shotter's references to 'sense' highlight how attuned responsiveness is not guaranteed: my felt sense of your feeling is already influenced by my own feelings and desires, making it possible that my declaration will be met with an awkward silence. However, if it turns out that our feelings are sufficiently shared, our future joint action will proceed more joyously. This dramatic example illustrates how, in relating, we constantly strive to anticipate each other's suggestions and concerns sufficiently for us to accommodate and negotiate them, and how we do this with reference to a mutually constituted, constantly unfurling background of feeling that sustains our conversation.

Although Langer's work does not contain any such detailed analyses, it is not fundamentally inconsistent with them. Writing about the evolution of language, for example, she first rejects suggestions that it was impelled by the desire for communication, since "There could hardly have been any desire or felt need to communicate among prehuman beings before there were definitely symbolic utterances to evoke ideas, associated with them by their producer" (Langer, 1972, p. 300). The desire to communicate already presumes a content it would seem useful to share: we could not want to share ideas expressible in language if we did not already have them. Instead, Langer's speculative account emphasises ritual, dance and other shared, rhythmic bodily activities, themselves organisations of "the need for contact between fellow creatures" (Langer, 1972, p. 311), and which – as epiphenomenon – engendered occasions or events for which names and categories might become functional. Hence, as language evolved:

> Its motivation was not communication, but communion, though not the sheer desire for bodily contact or at least intimate nearness of ape and monkey bands; what found expression in the dance was the sense of a power residing in the horde as a single agent, pervading the holy place and perhaps made visible in a fetish – a mysterious central tree or a nearby, terrible 'bush-devil', made by nature as a chance form, or by primitive but fantasy-guided hands. The reason for formalising the expression of group feeling was that in this way it was enhanced, sustained and upheld when subjectively it might have breaks and lapses.
>
> (Langer, 1972, pp. 301–302)

So Langer argues that linguistic utterances originated in collective dance rituals, communal organisations and incitements of feeling that could be extended and symbolically invoked when the shared, repetitive, rhythmic sounds accompanying them – patterns of breathing, grunting, squealing, stamping – were utilised on other occasions. This was only possible precisely *because* these sounds already had shared meanings derived from their status as prior elements of collective ritual. Protohumans thus had a mode of relating that was communal, rather than social, grounded in excitability and experiential empathy rather than sympathy or reflection – a mode visible today in flocks of birds, schools of fish and herds of deer. For Langer it was the recurrence in this communal mode of shared occasions of embodied being-with, rather than any putative desire to talk, that impelled the evolution of language.

It is a relatively short conceptual distance from the claim that communal organisations of feeling facilitated the evolution of language to Shotter's explorations of how emergent organisations of shared feeling support everyday discursive interaction. Moreover, the communal, sustaining and transformative functions of embodied being-with remain important today (Ehrenreich, 2007). Amongst the masses gathered at football stadiums, music festivals or political demonstrations, communication and togetherness frequently include a kind of pre-reflective carnal relationality, where common bonds are enacted through shared movement and gesture: the ritualised chants of football supporters or political protestors, the rhythmic, mannered movements of dancers, the shared orientation to an iconic fetish – the team, the DJ or singer, the leader – towards which these are directed. Langer's work also contains other discussions of the sociality of animals that posit a role for autogenic feedback (i.e. one initial driver of activity might also be that it feels good for the animal) as well as emphasising communal, reproductive, nurturing and survival needs. Likewise, her brief discussions of psychoanalysis also show how she recognised the importance of social relations.

Nevertheless, just as sociology and social psychology frequently bracket off the biological and the embodied in order to bring social influence into sharper focus (Newton, 2003), so Langer frequently downplays the social to clarify how the feeling body constitutes experience. Perhaps, had Langer's intentions been realised, the third volume of *Mind* would have contained a more detailed consideration of human sociality. But unfortunately:

> the hindrances of age – especially increasing blindness – make it necessary to curtail the work at what should be its height and contract the end into no more than a sketch of its presumptive final section.
>
> (Langer, 1982, p. 201)

Langer's ageing body sabotaged her work, and she died just three years after the truncated third volume of *Mind* was published. Maybe the relative omission of contemporary human social relations in her work would have been addressed, or maybe her work would have resembled many philosophies in being insufficiently social. In what she did write, however, social influences were frequently de-emphasised, in favour of an evolutionary focus that in practice downplays modern human sociality. Consequently, Langer's account of feeling must be integrated with contemporary analyses of social and relational influence, and with accounts that allow the continual connections between the biological and the social to be made apparent. This is the task of the next two chapters.

# 3
# Relating

It can sometimes seem like nothing is more obvious than the brute fact of individuality. In Chapter 1, it was argued that psychology tends to enact a relatively sharp dualism between individuals and social relations, and this helps constitute the discipline. If taken to its logical conclusion, this tendency becomes individualism, a moral and political stance prioritising individual rights, choices and interests over social needs, collective aims and shared interests. Individualism can be contrasted with collectivism, the stance that we are already interdependent, our well-being and survival necessarily dependent upon those of others. Individualism and collectivism have been studied cross-culturally, and it is generally accepted that English-speaking cultures are more individualist and Asian cultures (exemplified by Japan, Pakistan and China) are more collectivist (Triandis et al., 1986).[1] Nevertheless, people vary in the extent to which they endorse locally dominant values: some from collectivist cultures are relatively individualist, and vice versa. Moreover, collectivist values are also endorsed by individualists, albeit at lower levels (Hui & Triandis, 1986). Absolute contrasts between individualism and collectivism are therefore unsustainable.

In psychology, the dualism between individual and society frequently maps onto the Cartesian dualism between mind and body. Psychology primarily treats bodies and brains as individual matters, on the presumption that social and cultural influence ends at the barrier of the skin. Consequently, the body typically appears in psychology as "the sexless hull of the robomind" (Stam, 1998, p. 4), a meat machine with no intrinsic connections with social and relational influences. Consequently, this chapter begins with a discussion of the biological body that demonstrates how it is already open to social influence. Some of the ways in which social and cultural influences upon bodies and feeling have been explored within the disciplines of social theory, sociology and social psychology will then be reviewed. This paves the way for an explanation of the ways in which feelings are for the most part already social (bound up with current social situations and responsive to them) and socialised (shaped with the impress of prior social relations and experience).

## The biological body

Since it is impossible to review all the evidence demonstrating that the biological body is continuously open to social, cultural and material influences, I will briefly consider two areas: neuroscience and epigenetics. As I have already suggested, whilst neuroscience is relevant to many of the arguments in this book, there is a danger of overstating its implications. Considered more broadly, however, its findings do suggest some important general conclusions about the mutually responsive associations between brain, body and social relations.

One influential study imaged the brains of London taxi drivers (Maguire et al., 2000), who must demonstrate an understanding of its complex road systems ("the knowledge") to gain their licence. Spatial memory is at stake here, for which the hippocampus is known to be important, and structural MRI scanning demonstrated that drivers had significantly larger posterior hippocampi than matched controls. It also found a dose–response relationship between hippocampal size and years spent taxi-driving, suggesting that taxi-driving caused the hippocampus to increase in size (rather than people with larger hippocampi preferentially gaining licences).

Another study, using fMRI, showed that regular piano practice increased patterns of activation in sensori-motor areas associated with fingers and hands, and the more that participants practised the greater the increase in activation. A further stage of the experiment asked some participants to stop physically practising piano, but to spend time everyday *imagining* doing so. Analyses demonstrated that participants in this condition showed comparable increases in activation to those who continued to practise physically (Bangert & Altenmueller, 2003).

Contemporary neuroscience has produced quite literally hundreds of these kinds of findings, all demonstrating how one or another brain region, structure or system responds differentially to stimuli, practices and events: in other words that, to a considerable extent, the brain is plastic. They are paralleled by research demonstrating that levels of hormones and neurotransmitters in the body and brain are responsive to external influences. Coates and Herbert (2008) showed that stockbrokers experienced raised testosterone after deals were successful and suggested that this could make them more aggressive and reckless in subsequent trading. Other research shows that when parents cuddle babies, beta-endorphin is released in the orbitofrontal region of the baby's brain, and dopamine is released in the brainstem and migrates to frontal areas. Conversely, babies parented by unresponsive carers typically have lower levels of dopamine and norepinephrine (Jones et al., 1997), and when left to cry their cortisol levels rise significantly (Gunnar & Donzella, 2002).

Taken together, such research demonstrates that whilst the gross structure of the brain is relatively stable, its fine structure – the neural networks, patterns of activation and relative size of different areas – are constantly being refashioned by external influences. Similarly, the biochemical milieu of hormones, neurotransmitters and peptides that bathes body and brain is continuously responsive to events and relations. The brain is not plastic without limit: whilst many stroke patients make good recoveries, for example, others experience significant lasting impairment. Pronouncements of plasticity are sometimes ideologically inflected (Pitts-Taylor, 2010) and misleading about what the evidence – taken in its totality – actually shows. At the same time, the degree of plasticity revealed in recent studies exceeds, and therefore challenges, the reductive, deterministic assumptions historically associated with biological research. Brain function is critically dependent upon both its fine structure and its biochemical milieu, and both are exquisitely responsive to social, material and relational influences.

Neuroscience is informed by the other biosciences, including genetics and epigenetics. Genetics has changed somewhat since the Human Genome Project showed that we have far fewer genes than expected (20,000 to 25,000, as opposed to over 100,000). Craig Venter, leader of the privately funded 'Celera' sequencing project, expressed the issue succinctly: "We simply do not have enough genes for this idea of biological determinism to be right ... The wonderful diversity of the human species is not hard-wired in our genetic code. Our environments are critical" (McKie, 2001). Venter's comments gave further impetus to an already-emerging interest in the environmental processes that regulate gene expression: epigenetics. Epigenetics[2] studies processes such as methylation, acetylation, phosphorisation and RNA interference that can have the effect of either silencing or amplifying gene expression, for example through histone modification (changes in the ways in which DNA sequences are stored, coiled and packed in the cell nucleus) that, effectively, make genes more or less available.

It is too early to make strong claims about how epigenetic processes shape psychological experience. Whilst there is an exponentially growing strand of epigenetic research in mental health, it has yet to attain the maturity and sophistication that would enable it to produce valid, generalisable findings. Moreover, most research funding for epigenetics is being channelled into physical illnesses, especially cancer. The significance of epigenetics therefore lies less in the claims it currently makes than the shift of focus it represents. Increasingly, geneticists do not see genes as acting in isolation: they see them as always acting in the context of specific environments, and their expression as always regulated by the characteristics of those environments.

This understanding challenges claims that there are single 'genes for' many attributes, that human abilities consist solely of encapsulated 'modules' preserved since the Pleistocene, or that we are the puppets of 'selfish' genes striving blindly to reproduce. As biologist Steven Rose (1997) observes, humans are complex, multi-cellular creatures who reproduce systemically and interdependently: the ability of any gene to replicate depends upon the survival and reproductive success of the individual of which it is an element. Simultaneously, amongst humans individual survival is partially dependent upon that of groups and collectives. So the notion that genes function selfishly to pursue their own reproduction is mistaken: human evolutionary selection occurs at the level of the organism (and perhaps beyond), not the gene.

Rose (1997) also explains how the popular idea of genes as discrete, stable biological entities is contradicted by cell biology. Cell nuclei contain many sequences of seemingly redundant DNA, and the sequences we call genes are frequently dispersed widely across chromosomes. When cells reproduce, these sequences get spliced and edited in ways that can create significant variation: effectively, many genes get 'assembled' from alternative DNA sequences. These processes of splicing and editing mean that the DNA sequences we call genes can 'jump', or move to other areas of the chromosome. Until the 1980 this jumping was thought extremely rare, but research now shows it to be quite common. Rose describes how these processes of splicing, editing and jumping are open to environmental influence because genes replicate within the environment of cells, themselves sitting within wider environments that modulate their activity: in this way, each instance of replication is modulated by environmental influence.

So both neuroscience and epigenetics demonstrate that, even at the level of genes, cells, neurons, hormones and neurotransmitters, external influence does not end at the skin. The embrained body is not some pristine nucleus of individuality, and the genetic template upon which it gets assembled is not wholly determinate. This certainly does not mean that genes have no influence, or that the brain is infinitely malleable. It simply demonstrates that biological influences are always already bound up with environmental influences, rather than being opposed to and operating separately from them. When babies develop in the womb, each instance of cell replication is regulated by tiny variations in local levels of available oxygen and nutrients. This is why even genetically identical twins have different fingerprints, and even at birth are not usually *so* identical that those who know them well cannot tell them apart. The embrained body is always in the world, and the brain is a continuously biosocial organ. Together, they form a system of systems that is continuously responsive, both to relatively concrete influences such as diet and trauma, and more intangible influences such as social status and the meanings of relationships. The biological body is *already* simultaneously a social body.

## The social body

This section will review some of the ways in which the body has been conceptualised and studied in social science, and which considers how the ways we use, hold and experience our bodies are inflected by social relations and the cultural norms and expectations they carry, and thus begins to show how feelings are shaped by, and responsive to, situations, relationships and experiences. Social scientific work on the body frequently adopts a phenomenological perspective that explores lived embodiment, the kinds of experience the body enables. It will be useful to begin this review by considering some classic work suggesting that sociological variables such as socio-economic status (SES) and gender have corresponding bodily signatures.

### SES and gender

With respect to SES and embodiment the work of Pierre Bourdieu has been highly significant. Bourdieu argued that experience is shaped by normative sets of bodily dispositions. A disposition is a socially acquired way of using, holding and relating to the body, whether of preference or taste or a habitual manner of standing, walking, gesturing or using the head or arms, all of these "always associated with a tone of voice, a style of speech and (how could it be otherwise?) a certain subjective experience" (Bourdieu, 1977, p. 87). Dispositions cluster into enduring patterns, and a cluster or pattern of dispositions is called a habitus.

A habitus inevitably reflects a social class position, and is therefore "political mythology realised, em-bodied, turned into … a durable manner of standing, speaking, and thereby of feeling of thinking" (op. cit., pp. 93–94).

The habitus functions as a 'structured structuring structure'. First, this means that the habitus is *structured* by prior experience: the pattern of acquired dispositions will reflect locally dominant norms. Second, the habitus is then *structuring*: acquired dispositions shape the world as we subsequently experience it, leading us to favour some possibilities and disregard others. And third, the habitus is a *structure*, since the dispositions of which it consists 'hang together' in ways that reflect social positions, forming relatively stable patterns that are recognisable indices of status and cultural location. Consequently, SES is not solely a matter of occupation, postcode or other material markers: it gets quite literally embodied in habitual movements, styles and codes, of which accents are perhaps the most obvious. The habitus similarly contains tastes and styles that imbue experience with boundaries and potentials, rendering some possibilities largely unthinkable and 'not for the likes of us', whilst making others seem desirable and 'natural'.

Similarly, Iris Marion Young's (1990) classic essay "Throwing Like a Girl" explored reasons why, on average, girls might learnt to throw differently to boys. Young summarises research showing that, in Anglo-American cultures at least, girls typically throw without fully extending their arms or twisting their bodies, they "do not reach back, twist, move backward, step, and lean forward. Rather, the girls tend to remain relatively immobile except for their arms, and even the arms are not extended as far as they could be" (Young, 1990, p. 145). She reflects upon this finding, noting that typical anatomical or physiological explanations (girls are weaker, shorter, have different brains, different proportions, or breasts that would obstruct vigorous arm movements) lack empirical support. Rather, Young argues, gendered upbringing practices inculcate specific styles of relating to and using the body, styles she characterises as either feminine or masculine. These practices include gender differences in the organisation of play and sport; the promotion of specifically 'feminine' ways of standing, walking, sitting, dressing and talking; and emotional norms which emphasise female caring and nurturing and attach greater anxiety and danger to girls' activities.

Young argues that these practices generate a feminine body style composed of three gendered modalities of experience: ambiguous transcendence (more so than men, women typically experience their bodies as both vehicle for potential action and as burden or obstacle); inhibited intentionality (women more typically experience their bodies as both capable and incapable, and this experience inhibits actual movement); and discontinuous unity (women are more likely to experience their bodies fragmentarily, capable and powerful only partially, or in certain situations). Consequently, Young suggests, women's use of the objective, geometric spaces they occupy tends – by comparison to men's – to be more hesitant and inhibited, since their experience of those spaces is structured by these three inhibiting, fragmenting modes of motility and emotionality. Simultaneously, Young is clear that these masculine and feminine styles are socially produced, not biologically determined. They generate 'on average' differences not necessarily tied to biological sex: hence, we have both masculine girls and feminine boys.

Both Young and Bourdieu have inspired empirical research that supports their claims. Allen (2004) showed how differences in the ways visually impaired children adapt to and resist the limitations of their impairment were related to differences in SES. His analysis demonstrated how "the socioeconomic conditions in which the habitus is formed influence how 'bodily possibilities' are perceived and managed, and thus whether resistance to the embodiment of disability and socio-spatial exclusion occurs" (op. cit., p. 503), resulting in a geographical space that, for the more privileged, was experienced as more extensive and accessible. Similarly, Fredrickson and Harrison (2005) operationalised Young's claims about feminine body style by showing that increases in self-objectification (engineered by allowing participants to view themselves in a mirror) produced greater decreases in motor performance at a throwing task for females than for males.

The analyses by Bourdieu and Young share some important elements: both emphasise the role of early experience; both emphasise the unnoticed, and sometimes unintentional, bodily effects of various forms of instruction; and both emphasise how acquired bodily influences operate pre-reflectively to shape choice, activity, deliberation and reflection in ways not readily apparent. Both describe the acquisition of what we can call somatic repertoires – of posture, gesture, preference, movement and feeling – that pre-exist acts of rational deliberation. Since these repertoires operate on the fringes of awareness and do not require deliberate reflection to be activated, they are relatively intransigent, enduring and transposable across different settings. In Bourdieu's words:

> The principles em-bodied in this way are placed beyond the grasp of consciousness, and hence cannot be touched by voluntary, deliberate transformation, can't even be made explicit; nothing seems

more ineffable, more incommunicable, more inimitable, and, therefore, more precious, than the values given body, made body by the
transformation achieved by the hidden persuasion of an implicit
pedagogy, capable of instilling a whole cosmology, an ethic, a meta-
physic, a political philosophy, through injunctions as insignificant as
'stand up straight' or "don't hold your knife in your left hand".

(Bourdieu, 1977, p. 94)

### Determinism, agency and consciousness

Every analysis has some cost: each interpretation displaces or negates
alternatives, and phenomena visible at one scale simply dissolve at
others. Bourdieu and Young identified how gross differences in social
practice might impact upon experience by forming generalised somatic
repertoires associated with broad sociological categories: but in doing
so they necessarily glossed over and aggregated significant nuance
and variation. Reflecting on her earlier essay, Young (1998) wrote that
she wished she had placed more emphasis on the positive aspects of
feminine body styles. Evaldsson (2003) showed how feminine body
styles are cross-cut by other influences, including SES and ethnicity.
Her study of a Swedish playground, which identified girls orchestrat-
ing boy's activities and using full-body throwing to score points in a
game, demonstrated significant variation in the extent to which gendered embodiments reflected the styles Young identified. Throop and
Murphy (2002, p. 196) suggest that Bourdieu's analysis reifies habitus
as "an almost palpable entity... a *thing* that does something", rather
than a continuous process of practice, improvisation and reflection.
Mutch (2003) contrasted Bourdieu's notion of habitus as a structure
that generates practice with the idea of a 'community of practice' from
which structures emerge. His study of public house managers identified
two different groups of managers (one described as traditional working
class, another described as more heterogeneous and more often female)
for whom the relations between structure and practice seemed to differ. And, taking a slightly different tack, Skeggs (2004) suggests that
Bourdieu pays insufficient attention to affect and feeling, and the ways
in which SES and gender identities intersect. She argues that both are
held in place by 'affective reproduction': the imposition and exchange
of feelings of abjection and shame within relational processes that legitimate gendered middle-class identities by systematically devaluing those
less fortunate.

Two interlinked concerns emerge from this literature: determinism,
and agency. The charge, levelled especially against Bourdieu (see e.g.

Shusterman, 1999), is that his conceptual framework is deterministic, takes insufficient account of variation, and downplays individual capacities for choice or agency. Moreover, as Skeggs (2004) implies, to the extent that emotion and feeling are discussed, their intricacies, reciprocities and exchanges are rarely detailed and homogenising perspectives predominate. Thus, because the somatic repertoires Bourdieu and Young posit can be acquired and influential without conscious guidance, they might seem to imply universal processes operating in a behavioural manner that largely eludes reflection and rationality.

There is a raft of complex issues here. Individual life trajectories are clearly not wholly determined by habitus and situation: Bourdieu himself was the son of a working class farmer and postal worker from a village in the French south. At the same time, evidence from psychology and neuroscience suggests that much human activity is indeed habitual, and many decisions are made without 'rational' consideration of the antecedent influences and situational cues prompting them (Kahneman, 2012), and it is simply improbable that environments and cues related to SES and gender do not figure within this habitual or unthinking activity.

To some extent these debates may reflect an elision between description and proscription, between identifying how things are and proclaiming how they should be: few would *want* to be determined by occult influences from their pasts. They may also reflect contemporary ideological pressures and parallel academic fashions[3] that emphasise individual choice and that downplay similarity in favour of celebrations of difference.[4] As Chapter 2 emphasised, another consideration is that agency and rationality are never solely the product of logical deliberation anyway: they also depend upon felt influences that constitute and 'pre-load' or filter the field of choices we encounter.

In any case, the somatic repertoires Bourdieu and Young identify are best understood as modal tendencies rather than behavioural certainties. Young was absolutely clear that the gendered embodiments she identified have an 'on average' character, and that neither is the exclusive property of its respective gender. Whilst neither she nor Bourdieu engaged extensively with developmental psychology, research there demonstrates that influences associated with SES and gender are always refracted through the particular relationships, family circumstances and experiences of individuals (Kagan, 1998). Variation is therefore inevitable, reflective of the contingencies and excesses of everyday life and the fluctuating vagaries of which it is constituted. Hence it is noteworthy that – unusually, for someone of his background – Bourdieu's father strongly encouraged him to better himself and pursue the best educational opportunities available.

These concerns lead to an even more fundamental issue: our understanding of consciousness. If agency, choice and reflection are always in part predicated upon embodied, pre-reflective influences, the nature and role of consciousness itself comes into question. As Throop and Murphy (2002, p. 195) put it:

> Bourdieu holds...that it is seldom the case that action stems from conscious, intentional, or reflective reference to motivations or 'projects' since most action is more accurately generated by a 'practical feel', or a habituated automaticity that is the antithesis of conscious reflection.

At stake is the extent to which consciousness controls activity, the extent to which we are rational choosers, able to reflect accurately and make fully informed choices, and the extent to which we have privileged insight into our own motives and experiences. Moreover, buried within these questions are other concerns about the extent to which feelings and emotions are already intentional and meaningful, versus the extent to which they require prior cognitive appraisal for their significance (Leys, 2011). Psychology has long adopted conflicting stances to these questions. Whilst psychoanalysis and behaviourism were strikingly different enterprises, both emphasised influences beyond awareness: the unconscious, and the environment. Humanistic psychology, by contrast, emphasised insight, awareness, and a self that could be sensibly comprehended and deliberately worked upon. The debate between Zajonc (1980, 1984) and Lazarus (1982) about the relationship between affect and cognitive appraisal remains unresolved, but mostly seems to have hinged upon the adoption of broader and narrower definitions of these phenomena. Unsurprisingly, then, contemporary psychology embraces all possibilities. Many studies use self-report measures, implying a consciousness with at least partial insight into its own workings. Simultaneously, other studies implicate structures of beliefs – schema – that lie below conscious reflection, whilst yet other studies within the implicit association paradigm treat self-reports with explicit mistrust.

At this point it will help to recall the discussion of feeling in the previous chapter. Although feeling is the most basic constituent of experience, the raw material from which all psychological categories are in part differentiated, it is also a-representational and ineffable. Its influence is known immediately and experientially, and often quickly forgotten unless seized upon and represented with language or other symbols. This already suggests a view of consciousness where insight is necessarily limited, a view of 'rational' choice as already shaped and guided by felt influences we might not be able to readily articulate, or indeed control. Moreover, feelings are responsive to social and relational influences – in the present, and from the past – of which we may not be entirely aware: we might know *how* we feel, but simultaneously struggle to understand why we feel as we do. This does not mean we are entirely without insight, and certainly does not mean that our actions are irrational in that they lack all sense and purpose. However, it does suggest a view of consciousness that is more layered and nuanced, and less comprehensive and accurate, than some perspectives allow.

## The psychological body

So the body – whether considered biologically or experientially – is already also a social body. With these conclusions in mind, this discussion of the psychological body begins by reflecting upon an iconic experiment: Schacter and Singer's (1962) study of emotion and its relation to cognition. Like only a small handful of studies in psychology this experiment is well-known beyond as well as within the discipline, and continues to be cited today in the context of arguments for the dominance of cognition. Some critical reflection upon its conduct and findings is therefore appropriate.

Although typically portrayed as a cognitive study, Schacter and Singer's experiment also considered social influences and – like all psychology experiments – its actual conduct was permeated and made possible by networks of social relations. In this experiment, three groups of participants were injected with epinephrine (adrenalin), whilst a fourth was injected with saline solution. However, all four were told they were being injected with a vitamin compound, 'Suproxin', and that the experiment was assessing its effects on vision. Of the three groups that received epinephrine, one was informed correctly about its effects (described as side effects of Suproxin); another was misinformed (being told that they might experience itching, numb feet or headaches); and the third was kept ignorant of any effects. After the injections an actor came into the room, pretending to be another participant, and followed one of two scripts. In the angry script he expressed growing irritation and eventual outrage at the items on a questionnaire; in the euphoric script he threw paper aeroplanes, built towers from manila folders and played with hula hoops left in the corner. The experimenters assessed the extent and manner of the participants' emotional responses to this actor: these assessments were the primary dependent variables.

Initial analysis showed that the adrenaline injection increased sympathetic nervous system activity in most participants (a few showed no measurable effect). Analysis of group differences in responses to the actors showed that participants who were either misinformed or ignorant about the effects of the injection (in the anger condition, for what are described as 'pragmatic reasons', the misinformed group was omitted) responded with significantly greater levels of either euphoria or anger, whereas both the placebo and the correctly informed groups showed less. In respect of euphoria these differences were visible on both self-report and behavioural indices (assessed by an observer through a two-way mirror). In respect of anger only the behavioural indices showed significant effects, a difference attributed to the participants' reluctance to display anger towards the experimenters – who, it is revealed, were also their lecturers.

Schacter and Singer interpreted their findings as showing that "by manipulating the cognitions of an individual in such [an aroused] state, we can manipulate his feelings in diverse directions" (op. cit., p. 395). They made this claim on the basis that, whereas significant increases in euphoria and anger were observed in the two groups not expecting to experience arousal, this did not occur for the group who were *correctly* informed about the effects of injection: "In the anger condition, such subjects did not report or show anger; in the euphoria condition, such subjects reported themselves as far less happy than subjects with an identical body state but no adequate knowledge of why they felt the way they did" (op. cit., p. 396). Therefore – and with reference to other studies, whose findings they summarise – the authors concluded that "Given a state of sympathetic activation for which no immediately appropriate explanation is available, human subjects can be readily manipulated into states of euphoria, anger and amusement. Varying the intensity of sympathetic activation serves to vary the intensity of a variety of emotional states" (op. cit., p. 396).

Whilst this conclusion actually contains two distinct and logically unconnected elements, subsequent summaries have typically reported only the first and the study is commonly said to demonstrate that emotion consists of undifferentiated arousal that depends upon cognitive cues for its interpretation (e.g. as either euphoria or anger). However, the alternative interpretation – suggested by the second element of this conclusion – is that chemically induced arousal magnifies the feelings generated by stimuli, but this effect is modulated by the presence or absence of knowledge about its cause. That is, *all* participants experienced feelings in response to the actors; those who received epinephrine tended to have more intense feelings. However, those who knew they had received a stimulant were able to discount its effects. Rather than demonstrate that emotion consists of undifferentiated arousal that requires cognitive interpretation for its meaning, then, the experiment might simply have demonstrated the unsurprising finding that feelings can be enhanced by drugs – especially when their effects are unknown.

This interpretation gains further support from an aspect of the findings that has since received little attention. Schachter and Singer's theory predicted that levels of emotionality should follow a definite sequence: participants deliberately misinformed about the drug effects should show the greatest emotional responses, followed by those kept ignorant of any effects. The emotional responses of those informed correctly about the drug effects should be lower than both of these groups, and equal to the emotional responses of those given the saline placebo. These predictions were confirmed for the first two groups: those misinformed about the side effects showed the largest responses, followed by those who were told that there were no side effects. However, rather than the two remaining groups being equal, the placebo group consistently showed *higher* responses than the group who were correctly informed about the effects of the drug. Commenting on this, the authors candidly observe that "[t]his is a particularly troubling pattern for it makes it impossible to evaluate unequivocally the effects of the state of physiological arousal, and indeed raises serious questions about our entire theoretical structure" (op. cit., p. 393). This failure of their results to follow the predicted pattern was even more troubling since "Though the emotional level is consistently greater in the Epi Mis[informed] and Epi Ign[orant] conditions than in the placebo condition, this difference is significant at acceptable probability levels only in the anger condition" (op. cit., p. 393). In other words, Schachter and Singer were initially able to achieve their headline result only in the angry condition – not in the euphoria condition.

They account for this failure on the basis that some participants in the groups who were misinformed about the injection might nevertheless have attributed their responses to its effects. Supporting this, they report comments from some participants in these groups, such as 'the shot gave me the shivers' ('shivers' being feelings on most interpretations, although the authors do not dwell on this). Hence they proposed that, for some participants, additional cognitions – inadvertently produced by the experiment itself – led to interpretations that undermined the design of their study: "the experimental procedure of injecting the subjects, by providing an alternative cognition, has, to some extent, obscured the effects of epinephrine" (op. cit., p. 394). They then conducted further analyses excluding those participants who, they said, demonstrated this effect. The remaining participants' responses were a closer match with their predictions, and it was these modified analyses which supplied their headline findings. Importantly, however, these exclusions and further analyses did not actually address the issue that the placebo group – who, according to the theory being tested, should not have shown *any* significant emotional response – did in fact respond emotionally. This further suggests that, instead of proving that emotion consists of undifferentiated arousal plus cognitive interpretation, the experiment merely showed that emotions can be modulated both by drugs and by knowledge of their effects.

Schacter and Singer's experiment is commonly said to provide evidence for the effects upon emotional experiences of cognitive interpretations: "by manipulating the cognitions of an individual ... we can manipulate his feelings" (op. cit., p. 395). Nevertheless, no cognitions were directly manipulated. Physiologically, Schachter and Singer manipulated participants with injections of either epinephrine or saline. Relationally, they manipulated participants by deceiving them about the content of the injections, then placing them into engineered and constrained social settings. The participants were deceived about the true purpose of the study, and the actors misleadingly presented as participants. Other social relations permeated the entire procedure and at points visibly influenced its results: recall that in the 'angry' condition self-report data did not follow the predicted pattern, a discrepancy attributed to reluctance by student participants to express anger towards lecturers. But, in all this, whilst cognitions were *presumed* to have been manipulated (and whilst participants' subjective experiences were no doubt influenced) there was no *direct* manipulation of cognitions, and no actual evidence that cognitions per se – conceptualised as discrete elements, separate and distinct from other aspects of experience – were independently influential. So despite its iconic status this experiment does not prove the cognitive influence it is said to demonstrate: indeed, it arguably did more to illustrate the conjoined power of social and biological influences. We might therefore conclude that its interpretation reflects its position within the emergent zeitgeist of cognitivism that, by 1962, was gathering momentum in psychology.

The rise of cognitivism also makes sense of a seeming paradox in respect of social psychology and the body. Historically, the body has long been relevant to social psychology, which studies how the presence of others influences us, emphasises the power of the situations where bodies are located, and has often focused upon phenomena – emotion, aggression, romantic relationships – to which bodies are necessarily relevant. Nevertheless, in recent decades social psychology has been largely concerned with cognition – whether social representations, social identities or social cognition generally – and as a consequence the body has largely disappeared. UK social psychology has also been considerably influenced by discursive psychology (Edwards & Potter, 1992), which treats cognition as occurring between rather than within individuals, and as enacted through conversation and interaction. Discursive psychology has many advantages over social cognitive approaches, especially because of its use of real life or naturalistic data, rather than data produced within artificial laboratory setups. Nevertheless, it shares with cognitive psychology a tendency to downplay the relevance of the body, and a relative disregard for embodiment (Cromby & Nightingale, 1999).

In recent years this psychological tendency has begun to dissipate, most obviously in relation to the emergent paradigms of embodied, embedded and situated cognition. Confusingly, not only do these paradigms overlap, they are also heterogeneous: for example, Wilson (2002) identifies six distinct strands within the embodied paradigm. The paradigms overlap because "Biological brains are first and foremost the control systems for biological bodies. Biological bodies move and act in rich real-world surroundings" (Clark, 1998, p. 506). Biological systems serve adaptive functions in actual environments; these systems therefore generate psychological experiences, and enable psychological processes, that reflect both the embodied character of these systems and their material and environmental situations. Cognition is always already embodied, embedded in ongoing activity, and situated in contexts, both material and social, that influence its course.

In this regard, an accelerating strand of social psychological research has begun to amass experimental evidence demonstrating that social influences are mediated and enabled by bodily systems. Whilst comprehensive integrative theories of embodiment in social psychology are lacking (Meier et al., 2012) empirical evidence is being generated in relation to numerous domains. Many studies, for example, show that during social interaction facial expressions become entrained with those of others (e.g. Bush et al., 1989), and some demonstrate entrainment in response to faces presented subliminally (Dimberg, Thunberg & Elmehed, 2000). Even reading can produce entrainment: Andersen, Reznik and Manzella (1996) used disguised versions of participants' own descriptions of significant others as the basis for fictional characters, and some while later mingled these with descriptions of other, wholly unknown characters. Participants were asked to read them all: when they did so, they exhibited more marked facial expressions – both positive and negative – in response to descriptions that evoked people they knew.

Other experiments show that connections between cognition and the body are not limited to facial expressions, and that body changes themselves seemingly produce feeling changes. These changes consist of experimentally malleable movement regimes with presumed affective connotations: approach movements that open the body to others are classed as positive, avoidance movements that close it or push others away are classed as negative; shaking the head is negative, whereas nodding is positive; and so on. For example, variations in body posture – sitting slumped or sitting upright – were shown to modulate reported feelings of pride following an achievement task (Stepper & Strack, 1993); participants viewing unknown Chinese ideographs whilst either pushing downwards on a table (avoidance) or upwards (approach) gave more positive affect ratings in the approach condition (Cacioppo, Priester, & Berntson, 1993); and participants asked to either shake or nod their heads – purportedly to check the fit of headphones – were more likely to choose as a gift a pen seen when nodding their heads, whereas those shaking their heads were more likely to choose a substitute gift (Tom et al., 1991).

Connections between the body and memory have also been shown using this headphone task. Participants were presented with lists of words, including some that were positively or negatively valenced. Participants nodding their heads demonstrated better recall for positively valenced words, whereas the opposite pattern was seen amongst participants shaking their heads (Forster & Strack, 1996). A recurrent theme in these experiments is compatibility: when body variables are compatible with the cognitive task (e.g. a hand movement approaching the body is paired with an affectively positive stimulus), the task is performed more rapidly, easily or efficiently. Conversely, when cognitive and body requirements are incompatible – for example, negatively valenced words are presented whilst facial muscles are producing a smile – performance is impaired.

Such evidence led Barsalou (1999) to challenge the view that concepts are abstracted, generalised representations not tied to sensory or bodily modalities, and so – like information processed within electronic media – their content does not influence their processing. On this view, the concept of anger, for example, is a generalised mental pattern or type composed of various, connected representations, against which individual instances or tokens of anger get compared.

Barsalou's alternative proposal is that conceptualisation is based upon enactment and simulation. Having the concept 'anger' means being able to integrate a learned pattern of modality specific elements – facial expressions, vocal intonations, postures, movements and subjective experiences – with the features of a given situation. From this perspective, we do not recognise anger by comparison with a store of abstract representations: we recognise it by conducting a set of partial re-enactments, the specific elements of which are prompted by features of the current situation as they relate to patterns arising on previous occasions. These simulations constitute a situated, embodied concept of anger that simultaneously includes the experiences of the person whose concept it is, and which is not dependent on separately stored representations:

> simulations of perception, action and introspection directly consti-
> tute the conceptual content of social knowledge. Knowledge is not a
> re-description of these states in an amodal language, but is the ability
> to partially re-enact them
>
> (Barsalou et al., 2003, p. 73)

Barsalou (1999) is explicit that, once understood as simulation and re-enactment, cognition does not only involve conscious processes. He notes evidence that many conscious processes are informed by and dependent upon non-conscious processes, so that "*Unconscious* re-enactments may often underlie memory, conceptualisation, comprehension and reasoning" (op. cit., p. 66). Although the evidence is tilted towards non-conscious processes, as a consequence of experiments within which participants are deflected from attending to the embodied processes being studied, "much evidence exists that embodiment effects result from automatic processes" (op. cit., p. 66).

Embodiment research in social psychology therefore converges upon similar concerns to those debated in social science.[5] Despite being guided by different theories, using different methods and reproducing different traditions, psychological research is also raising questions of consciousness, determinism and agency. Like Bourdieu and Young, psychological research recognises that influences can impinge upon us without our noticing, and that many of our responses are habitual. Whilst the findings of this research are broadly compatible with the argument that somatic repertoires associated with sociological variables are modal, 'on average' and probabilistic rather than deterministic, it pays little heed to SES and gender. Issues of determinism and agency nevertheless become relevant, because many studies seemingly demonstrate the effects of influences of which participants themselves appear unaware. So, whilst there are methodological issues which may lead us to question the validity and generality of specific experiments (see Chapter 5), discussions of this research nevertheless converge with related discussions in social science.

## The feeling body

This chapter has considered the body as it appears in biology, social science and psychology. From each perspective, there is good evidence that social, relational and material influences continuously shape embodied experience. Despite cultural tendencies that encourage us to experience our bodies as encased, hardened and separate there is evidence demonstrating that social and cultural influences permeate the ways we use, hold and experience our bodies, that they help constitute our tastes, preferences and desires, and that our biology is functionally responsive to their impingements. It is therefore to be expected that the process of feeling is also open to other processes that are more overtly social, cultural, relational and material. This can be explained with reference to the analytic classes of feeling set out previously.

Feelings of knowing are intrinsically social. They are always situated in and reflective of ongoing streams of activity which both incite them and lend them their full significance. Whether considered in their relational aspect, as providing knowledge about the momentary status and trajectory of an interaction, or in their intellectual aspect where they provide a felt response to a proposition, argument, claim or statement, feelings of knowing are thoroughly bound up with the ongoing concerns of the social and material world. As we have seen, Shotter (e.g. 1993a) provides an excellent account of their relational aspects, whilst Johnson (2007) supplies an insightful discussion of their intellectual dimensions.

Emotions are likewise social, in the sense that they are relational. Friends and lovers are those with whom we disclose feelings not acknowledged in other contexts, people with whom we share values and morals and can voice anxieties, desires and hopes: hence, the exchange and caring management of emotion is what in large part makes these relationships significant. This is why Burkitt's (2014) notion of emotions as relational complexes posits that emotions actually *constitute* social relations – as for example loving, impatient, trusting, suspicious, desiring, indifferent, caring or dismissive. In Burkitt's account emotions are not consequent upon individual cognitive interpretations: rather, emotions are aspects of, or elements within, lived dynamic social interactions. His concept of emotion – with which the notion of feeling advanced here has some parallels – views it as complex in three senses. First, emotions are intrinsically part of ensembles or patterns of relationships, where they continuously contribute to their qualities and dynamics. Second, emotions are themselves complex or complicated, their various psychological, physiological, neural and social elements combining so that "socially meaningful relationships register in our body-minds and, at some level of awareness, are felt" (Burkitt, 2014, p. 15). Third, emotions are complex in that they involve a pattern of relations, felt in a particular way, which arises along a continuum between being helplessly overcome by emotion at one end to being in control and finessing emotion at the other.

Burkitt (2014) further emphasises the social aspects of emotions by emphasising their historical and cultural specificity. Drawing on historical scholarship he traces romantic love back to traditions of courtship and adulation first associated with troubadours in the 12th century. Likewise, drawing on anthropological studies of maternal love and child death in a Brazilian shantytown, Burkitt shows how it is specific to its cultural and material situation, since mothers living in these desperately deprived, malnourished communities did not grieve for infants that died, only for their older children.

Emotional feelings are also socialised, and Ahmed's (2004) analyses demonstrate how they can be understood in relation to intersections of gender, race, class and sexuality that together constitute a dynamic cultural politics of emotion. Their enculturation is highlighted by research, mentioned previously, that demonstrates both historical and geographical variability between cultures with respect to the forms, significances and prevalence of emotion. Their socialisation is indexed by the ways in which they continuously get enrolled within, and become relevant for, social practices and situations. Hochschild's (1983) influential notion of emotional labour describes how, in accord with the demands of paid employment, workers must frequently manage their own emotions and those of others. Scores of studies have demonstrated how the demands of employment frequently include requirements to manage – produce, suppress, restrain, display – emotions in the self, and simultaneously manage – absorb, placate, control, appreciate, enjoy – the emotions of others. From fast-food workers wishing customers to 'have a nice day', through the expectation that sex workers' enjoy their clients desires and respond with apparently sincere feeling to their wishes (Sanders, 2005; Vanwesenbeeck, 2005), to the more subtle expectation that academics hide the emotional injuries their work inflicts in order to remain productive and reassure students (Gill, 2009; Parker, 2014), emotional or affective labour (Hardt, 1999) is central to our service-oriented economy.

Extra-emotional feelings, finally, are at least socialised, if not actually social: they bear the impress of prior experience, even if their current occurrence is seemingly prompted by events or stimulations experienced as wholly internal. Studies of pain – the extra-emotional feeling which might seem at first glance most purely biological or natural – reveal clear evidence of socialisation, understood in the sense of reflexive practice (deliberate, or incidental) within social settings and relationships, which modifies what is felt. Martial arts and military training include practices of hitting and being hit by others that, over time, make pain easier to both inflict and withstand, eventually lowering the threshold beyond which pain becomes incapacitating (e.g. Focht, Bouchard, & Murphey, 2000). Pain is also socialised in practices of sadomasochism, where it gets associated and combined with feelings of sexual pleasure and is reflexively worked on in pursuit of new, different or more intense experiences (Beckmann, 2001; Langdridge & Barker, 2007). In a more everyday fashion, pain is also socialised, implicitly and unintentionally, by the responses of parents and others to the many inevitable small physical injuries of childhood. In responding to children's pain, carers model how the child should respond, so communicating implicit feeling rules that become part of later experience: telling a child what to do is, simultaneously, telling her how to be (Shotter, 1989). These lines of influence are not homogenous so that gendered expectations, for example, are not always unequivocally transmitted; nevertheless, there is good evidence of family influences upon later experiences of chronic pain (Evans et al., 2008).

Socialisation is apparent in relation to other extra-emotional feelings. Hunger gets socialised differently between cultures, so that dishes deemed appetising by one culture – insects, hot spices, sea bird carcasses fermented in salt (an Innuit specialty) – are considered repulsive by others. Hunger also gets socialised *within* cultures, as people attend weight-management classes, engage with 'pro-ana' websites, restrain their eating or, alternately, enter into 'feeder' relationships that cultivate increased body mass (Monaghan, 2005; Mateus et al., 2008). Sexual desire, similarly, gets socialised differently between cultures: the modesty conferred upon Muslim women by the Hijab can seem wholly unnecessary to Anglo-American men, just as Anglo-American women visiting Islamic cultures can become inadvertent foci of the male gaze by dressing as they usually would. Christian cultures, meanwhile, hark back to the Adam and Eve myth both to render sexual desire dangerous and to associate it with stereotypical gender roles. Catholicism socialises sexual desire in relation to heterosexual marriage and reproduction, through strategies such as attaching guilt to masturbation, extra-marital sex and 'excessive' sexual pleasure, and until recently demanded even of married women who have given birth that they be 'churched' – that is, repent for having engaged in sexual activity – before again receiving communion (Davies, 2012).

## Conclusion

Feelings are enabled by the living body, and that body is always in a social and material world. Consequently, the feelings it supplies are infused with social and relational influence. Feelings primordially co-constitute experience, and our subjective grasp upon their intimate character and location can make them seem wholly our own. But many influences upon the ways that we feel lie far beyond the boundaries of our bodies, and for this and other reasons may not be readily grasped. Smail (1987, p. 71) describes how a conscientious, capable woman working with children in care felt guilty because she was unable to be profoundly moved by the children she worked with. After months of berating herself for her shame-inducing personal failing, one night she attended a parents' evening at a school. Waiting to speak with a teacher she was suddenly struck by the anxious concern of the mother in front, how "she felt worried about her daughter in a way which was simply not possible for someone whose interest in a child was merely professional". In Smail's clinical work with the woman, this incident helped her realise that whilst both her guilt and her caring were experienced as subjective feelings, they were constituted from social and material arrangements within which she was embedded and which she was largely powerless to change.

This chapter has described how evidence from the social sciences and from psychology converge to supply a view of bodies as the carriers of sometimes covert or unnoticed social influences. This poses questions about agency and determinism, and this undermines notions of consciousness as unitary and insightful. Somatic repertoires – gestures, postures, modes of comportment and bearing – are organised by cultural expectations and experienced in accord with normative requirements. Feelings of all kinds are similarly open to social influence and – at least, by the time, we can reflect upon them – are already to some extent socialised. Some implications of this for the ways that feelings constitute experience will be considered in the next chapter.

# 4
# Experiencing

This chapter will consider some of the relationships between feelings and experience. In recent years, there has been a small trend amongst psychologists to focus primarily upon experience itself, as opposed to focusing on the components (cognition, affect, memory, perception) from which it is constituted. Middleton and Brown (2005) study how experience is produced by dynamic processes of remembering. Drawing on Halbwachs and Bergson they argue against static, 'container' notions of memory, proposing instead that remembering continuously 'gnaws into the present'. The past is a virtual realm constantly getting actualised in the present, where its invocations co-constitute experience by giving it temporal direction and personal meaning. By contrast, Stephenson and Papadopoulos (2007) are more overtly concerned with power. They develop a post-Foucauldian notion of experience within which disciplinary practices continuously and contingently generate excesses that subvert their own force: this means that experience is always shaped by power relations, but never wholly determined by them. Taking another perspective, Bradley (2005) explores the relations between time, contingency and experience, drawing on psychoanalysis to understand some of the ways in which our experience of ourselves is always somewhat obscure and lacking transparency.

Whilst there are many differences between these substantial works, they all share an orientation towards experience as something to be explained. Rather than treat experience as some kind of transcendent origin (a stance associated with Cartesian dualism and individualism: Sampson, 1983) each explores some of the processes whereby experience is actually constituted. In examining how memories, power relations and temporal shifts lend experience its particular characteristics, they demonstrate how individual experience is formed in relays where it is always bound up with social structures, relational dynamics and material circumstances.

A similar strategy will be followed in this chapter, which will emphasise how experience is co-constituted by feelings and language. Experience will be conceptualised quite broadly as implying elements of the phenomena described by related terms such as mind, thought and consciousness. It will also be taken to imply notions of selfhood or subjectivity, aspects of experience which will receive explicit attention in relation to discussions of habit. The chapter begins, however, by briefly considering some of Langer's views on the significance of art.

## Art and language

Art is important for Langer because it is "the objectification of feeling" (Langer, 1967, p. 87): it makes concrete and tangible the experiential tensions, rhythms, patterns and textures of feeling that, because they are embodied and a-representational, cannot adequately be communicated using words or symbols. Music described as 'sad', for example, does not simply express the misery of the composer or player, who need not be feeling sad to write or perform it and might well find sadness a hindrance to doing so. Likewise, this music does not actually need to make listeners feel sad for them to recognise its affective intent. Therefore, what sad music does is not so much express or inculcate sadness as convey a sense or 'image' of how sadness feels. In its performance, it makes tangible some of the textures and dynamics of sadness, rendering them as recognisable analogues that convey a shared notion of that feeling.

On this basis, Langer argues that art serves two functions. The first is that

> it articulates our own life of feeling so that we become conscious of its elements and its intricate and subtle fabric, and it reveals the fact that the basic forms of feelings are common to most people at least within a culture.
>
> (Langer, 1967, p. 64)

So art permits a glimpse into the private realm of feeling experienced by others, allowing us to share something of its ineffable particularities. In this way, art also provides an evidence base demonstrating the generality and ubiquity of human feeling. If large numbers of people are seemingly moved in similar ways by a particular work, this suggests that these people share capacities to experience certain feelings.

The second function of art is that potentially lends new form or structure to felt experience, allowing us to interpret it anew. Illustrating this, Langer describes how abstract painting and constructivist sculpture developed in response to changing social standards and material circumstances, and how, once these forms developed, they acted back on the experience of those who made them:

> The power of abstraction became a central need, and the elimination of referential meaning threw the whole task of organising the work on the artist's imagination of sheer perceptual values. The great 'abstract' painters and constructivist sculptors are clearing the way to a new vision; and when they have found and completely mastered the principle of its presentation, they presumably will turn to nature again for the same purpose as before. And it will look different to their eyes.
>
> (Langer, 1967, p. 87)

Art is therefore both "the objectification of feeling, and the subjectification of nature" (Langer op. cit.). On the one hand, it renders visible the private rhythms and gradients of feeling; on the other, it educates the senses into novel perspectives upon the ways in which feeling already inhabits their products. This is possible because art creates both primary and secondary illusions. A painting in a gallery can create the primary illusion that a landscape lies before us. Simultaneously, the painting can create the secondary illusion that this landscape is imbued with movement, potential, growth, development, tension, that it is ominous, friendly, warm, cold, inviting, hostile, energetic, tired and so on. Thus, it is in secondary illusions that we 'see' in the perceptible world the movements of our own feelings.

It is by contrast with art that Langer discusses the very pinnacle of symbolisation: language. Language is massively significant in Langer's analysis of mind because it is "intrinsic to thinking, imagining, even our ways of perceiving" (Langer, 1972, p. 318), it penetrates absolutely all of our capacities to reason and act and in so doing "lifts them from their animalian state to a new, peculiarly human level" (op. cit., p. 324). Language is therefore absolutely critical for Langer's analysis, albeit not exclusively so: for her, experience is always thoroughly suffused by its categories and distinctions, even whilst she recognises that it never operates alone:

> The depth to which the influence of language goes in the formation of human perception, thought and mental processes generally

is as amazing as its evolution from human feeling, peripheral and central.

(Langer, 1972, p. 351)

Langer argues that the great strength of language is that it divides phenomena into discrete units that can be abstracted, generalised, manipulated, transformed and otherwise conceptually worked over or communicated. In this way language wields immense power in human life and is a crowning achievement of our species. Nevertheless, in order to coherently and sensibly derive these units:

> What can be stated has to be logically projectable in the discursive mode, divisible into conceptual elements which are capable of forming larger conceptual units somehow analogous to the concatenations of words in language.

(Langer, 1967, p. 102)

Language requires phenomena that can be meaningfully segmented into discrete units, designated using words or phrases arranged in a linear fashion. But feeling is not singular, discrete and sensibly divisible, its dynamics are not necessarily linear or sequential, and nor is it capable of straightforward representation. Hence, with respect to feeling – and by contrast with art – language becomes:

> clumsy and all but useless for rendering the forms of awareness that are not essentially recognition of facts, though facts may have some connection with them. They are perceptions of our own sensitive reactions to things inside and outside of ourselves, and of the fabric of tensions which constitutes the so-called 'inner life' of a conscious being. The constellations of such events are largely non-linear… and those which rise to a psychical phase – that is to say, felt tensions – can be coherently apprehended only in so far as their whole non-psychical organic background is implied by their appearance.

(Langer, 1967, p. 103)

So whilst Langer recognises the massive importance of language, with respect to feeling she is also acutely aware of its shortcomings: this makes it necessary to turn elsewhere for detailed discussion of its functions and effects. Whilst the decades since the linguistic turn (Harre, 1992) have generated masses of relevant psychological and social scientific research, the present focus on experience makes it appropriate to first consider Vygotsky's account of the origins of inner speech.

## Language and inner speech

Wertsch (1991) identifies three interwoven themes in Vygotksy's writings: genetic analysis, the dependence upon social relations of individual functioning, and an understanding of how action is mediated by tools and signs. Genetic analysis, here, means considering the origins and transitions that produce a phenomenon in its current form, since "it is only in movement that a body shows what it is" (Wertsch, 1991, p. 20). Whilst Vygotsky thought this mode of analysis applicable in domains including the phylogenetic and the historical or socio-cultural, he mainly applied it to psychological phenomena. Likewise, Vygotsky's interest in how 'higher mental functions' are *derived from* social relations – rather than simply contextually influenced by them – also exemplified his focus on the psychological. His concern with mediation and how activity gets transformed by the inclusion of tools or signs was similarly most evident in relation to psychological questions, particularly about how children learn. This psychological and applied emphasis reflects the situation of Vygotsky's work in Soviet Russia following the 1917 revolution, where he contributed to the massive programme of education initiated by the Bolsheviks.

Vygotsky's account of the development of inner speech exemplifies how these three themes infuse his work. A particular concern is the phenomenon of children speaking aloud to themselves whilst learning. It is well known that Piaget described this as 'egocentric speech' and treated it as relatively unimportant: for him, it reflected the child's self-centred failure to recognise that such talking is disruptive to others, and its gradual disappearance signalled a growing awareness of the needs of others. In contrast, Vygotsky saw this kind of talking – which is more sensibly called outer speech – as evidence of learning. He proposed that outer speech is actually a transitional form, halfway between the conversation it was derived from and the inner speech it will become. Conversations, especially in instructional settings, provide templates for later self-directed activity. When learning a task we often 'replay' fragments of these conversations by speaking them aloud. As competence grows this happens less, but the conversations remain influential in the form of silent, unspoken inner speech: a running commentary on experience that supplies metacognitive tools to monitor and guide activity.

Vygotsky formulated this claim explicitly in his 'general genetic law of cultural development':

> Any function in the child's cultural development appears twice, or on two planes. First it appears on the social plane, and then on the psychological plane. First it appears between people as interpsychological category, and then within the child as an intrapsychological category... Social relations or relations among people genetically underlie all higher functions and their relationships.
>
> (Vygotsky, 1978, p. 57)

This 'law' involves more than the mere truism that psychological processes develop within social relations. Vygotsky was making the stronger claim that the specific structures and contents of inner speech relate directly to the conversations from which it was derived. Whilst adults can struggle to appreciate this, many can use the example of driving: a skill typically learned relatively late in life and outside the family home, two factors that can make the origins of its associated inner speech more obvious. Faced with a complicated situation, drivers sometimes find themselves rehearsing phrases their driving instructor used in similar circumstances. They may do this aloud (Vygotsky showed this is more likely when tasks are demanding) or silently, but in each case it will be the instructor's words that get rehearsed – and most probably also their (hopefully calming) tone of voice. Such experiences illustrate the genetic connections between conversation, outer (egocentric) speech and inner speech; the development of individual psychological capacities by taking up elements from prior social relations; and the ways that (linguistic) tools mediate and transform psychological processes.

Vygotsky's account has limitations. Wertsch (1991) observes that Vygotsky overstated the significance of language, since evidence from cultures less reliant on verbal communication shows that psychological abilities can be mediated by visual and other means. Another concern is that Vygotsky posited the relative independence of biological and socio-cultural processes in infancy, claiming that they only come together later in development. This tendency towards dualism, which is visible elsewhere in his work (van der Veer & Valsiner, 1991) is challenged by studies of child development and interaction, and by neuroscientific research (Trevarthen & Aitken, 2001). Relatedly, some commentators have noted that Vygotsky's distinction between lower and higher mental functions is unclear (Meshcheryakov, 2007). Additionally, despite his emphasis upon socio-cultural influences, Vygotsky did not actually engage much with broader historical, institutional or cultural processes (Papadopoulos, 1996).

Notwithstanding these limitations, Vygotsky's work has been massively influential. Its initial importance lies in the way it subverts any sharp divide between individuals and social relations by showing that one of the most intimate and prominent elements of experience, inner speech, has social origins. However, it is also important because of its capacity to forge links with Langer's account of feeling. One of Vygotsky's best-known claims is that 'language completes thought',[1] a statement clearly demonstrating his recognition that thinking is not just unspoken conversational fragments. And thinking clearly does consist of more than words; sensory processes of seeing, hearing, smelling and tasting often contribute, whilst the complex processes of remembering are almost universally significant (Middleton & Brown, 2005). But in concluding his seminal work on thinking and speech, Vygotsky – like Langer – emphasises felt, bodily experience.

> Thought... is engendered by motivation, i.e. by our desires and needs, our interests and emotions. Behind every thought there is an affective-volitional tendency, which holds the answer to the last 'why' in the analysis of thinking.
>
> (Vygotsky, 1962, p. 150)

Thus, both Langer and Vygotsky see feeling as constitutive of experience, and both see it as coming before formal, logical or discursive influences.[2] Although social constructionism also emphasises language, relatively few constructionist writers engage directly with experience per se, tending to focus instead on the discourses and narratives that supply (some of) its conditions of possibility. However, Billig (1987) provided a scholarly account of thinking with interesting resonances with Vygotsky's. Billig argued that thought is dialogically structured – that it always bears the traces of possible counter-positions or arguments, which its formulation is already designed to refute. The similarity here is not just in the claim that thought is socially influenced, but that particular features of thought can be traced to specific aspects of social interaction. In a similar vein, dialogical self theory (Hermans, 2002) proposes that selves emerge in the tension between imagined subject positions in dialogue. This dialogue can be external or relational; internal, in the form of inner speech, or both. Like Mead, Hermans sees the self as a 'society of mind' populated by a multiplicity of relatively autonomous and sometimes conflicting "I" positions, reflective of our previous and current social engagements, which we occupy and 'speak from' in any given moment.

Analyses such as these have considerably extended our understanding of how language constitutes experience. Constructionist studies of discourse, rhetoric, conversation and naturalistic interaction, alongside empirical research modelled on the dialogical self, have made vital contributions to psychology and social science by demonstrating how the individual is interpenetrated by the social. At the same time, in almost exclusively emphasising language these analyses can leave little room for feeling. For example, Billig (1999) extended his study of the rhetorical character of thinking by showing how Freudian repression is learned in social interaction. In this important work Billig particularly emphasises 'little' words and innocuous phrases ('but', 'anyway', 'oh well') that can unobtrusively deflect conversation from one topic to another. Freud never explained how repression is learned, and Billig proposes that its origins are in social interaction: we learn to repress in thought just as, in conversation, we learn to avoid difficult topics. Whilst this is a valuable insight, Billig does not theorise the toxic feelings which typically serve as motivation or target for these repressive dialogues. Following Wittgenstein he argues that emotions are not just inner states but also social accomplishments, yet in so doing renders them largely devoid of any relationally significant bodily aspects. Consequently, whilst recognising its strengths and insights, reviewers judged his version of repression a sanitised one where the everyday needs, unspeakable desires and dangerous motivations of the body are largely invisible (Wortham, 2001) and which does not consider the feelings, particularly shame, with which repression is associated (Scheff, 2000).

Similarly, notwithstanding attempts to identify its neural basis (Lewis, 2002) and an intellectual lineage that includes Bakhtin, the dialogical self is, in practice, largely disembodied. Although empirical studies explore constellations of subject positions associated with (i.e. embodied within) particular individuals, the dialogues between these positions are conceived of as almost exclusively linguistic, such that the feelings Langer and Vygotsky saw as underpinning all dialogue are rarely if ever explicitly considered. Dialogue occurs between narrated subject positions rather than from within a more inchoate pulsing of sometimes contradictory felt impulses, and language does not complete thought so much as largely encompass it. Consequently, the dialogical self is overly rational, tends towards linguistic determinism, and effectively conceives of selfhood in terms of discordant subject positions that are symbolised and represented rather than lived and experienced.

## Language and feeling

Bringing together the lines of argument proposed by Langer and Vygotsky suggests a notion of experience as a continuous process of feeling, which gets seized upon by language, which impels feeling and so on. Relatedly, Langer emphasises an interplay between the objectification of feeling (which, for her, often means art) and the subjectification of nature, the endowment of natural forms with felt import, proposing that "[t]he dialectic of these two functions is, I think, the process of human experience" (1967, p. 241). Thus, for Langer the dynamics of language and inner speech are already inhabited by, and, to a lesser extent, directive of, embodied dynamics of feeling and perception. The occasional moments where we are either lost for words or, conversely, do not quite know how to feel, both reveal the continuous operation of this felt dialectic and, simultaneously, show how experience is profoundly enrolled within sometimes contradictory norms, unsayable claims or normatively excessive feelings.

Experience in this sense (and others – Stephenson & Papadopoulos, 2007) is continuous: nevertheless, we can further illuminate some of its movements by artificially breaking its processes into discrete moments, many of which – in Langer's terms – could be conceived of as *acts*. In Langer's philosophy, acts encompass a wide range of seemingly disparate phenomena, from reflex actions, salivation, heartbeats and the firing of a neuron, right through to more complex phenomena such as aggression towards authority figures. What these all share, Langer argues, is a temporal form consisting of a phase structure that typically includes incipience, acceleration and consummation, and then cadence or diminution (Langer, 1967, pp. 288–289). Acts, therefore, are spatio-temporally organised sequences of living processes. They always occur within given situations that prompt them, situations that include both the external, material environment and "the constellation of other acts in progress" (Langer, 1967, p. 281). Acts emerge as distinguishable dynamic patterns within the ongoing activity of living creatures, where

> [t]hey normally show a phase of acceleration, or intensification of a distinguishable dynamic pattern, then reach a point at which the pattern changes, whereupon the movement subsides. The point of general change is the consummation of the act.
>
> (Langer, 1967, p. 261)

A first point of consummation, then, is when inner speech functions to isolate and stabilise elements of the flux of feelings that constitute experience, acting to 'complete' and therefore subtly transform them. In Shotter's (1993b) terms, inner speech functions to make feeling intelligible, as opposed to merely meaningful. This enables us to represent to ourselves and others our felt desires and needs, and so achieve a more intersubjective or conventionalised knowledge of our own experience.

Second, inner speech can provoke feeling. We might, for example, find ourselves 'replaying' criticisms by an anonymous reviewer of a paper we submitted, whilst simultaneously experiencing many toxic feelings (cf. Gill, 2009), in an almost instantaneous dialectic where inner speech provokes feelings that are rapidly 'completed', provoking further feelings which (almost) immediately provoke others. 'Dialectic' here implies a flux of mutually constitutive movements of realisation and suppression (in Hegelian terms, a sublation): not a jarring or clashing opposition. Consequently, feelings and inner speech are typically enmeshed and concordant – such that when occasionally they are not we tend to notice this as we might, for example, attempt to 'talk ourselves into' doing whatever our feelings disbar.[3]

Third, both feelings and inner speech are mutually constitutive of social interaction, which in turn constitutes modes of experience: that is, there is a simultaneous dialectic within the associations between experience and ongoing social relations. Mutually worked-up feelings guide conversations, such that how we relate and what we experience are sensitively intertwined in processes of mutual becoming. Our utterances can therefore be characterised as 'rhetorical-responsive' (Shotter, 1993b). They are responsive to the dynamically co-created context into which they are spoken, and rhetorical because tailored in recognition of its imperatives and reflective of our attempts to move it along. Experience is consequently a 'boundary phenomenon' (Shotter, 1993c): neither simply 'inside' nor simply 'outside', but continuously re-created within ethically charged intersecting planes of feeling and language.

Fourth, this suggests a continuously liminal field of contingent experience, always stretched between the felt and the discursive, where feeling is constantly being provoked then represented by images and prompts generated both within the body and around it. These contingencies engender lines of differentiation that get dichotomised in our culture into two largely distinct categories. To the extent that feeling can be more-or-less entrained, completed by and symbolised within discursive practice, we categorise it largely as thought, reasoning or deliberation (in the process largely downplaying the distinctly somatic aspects of intellectual processes such as feeling curious, puzzled, confident or unsure). Conversely, to the extent that the velocities, movements and intensities of feeling exceed or outstrip the linear, sequential, segmenting capacities of language, or to the extent that its valences and textures are discordant with the normative expectations of our situation (broadly, the discursive forms we can legitimately deploy), we categorise it affectively, as emotion (in the process often downplaying the symbolic, performative, already-intentional aspects of these emotional feelings).[4]

And fifth, as the term 'dialectic' suggests, the bi-directional lines of influence between feeling and inner speech can produce something qualitatively new. Vygotsky (1962) showed how the transformation from outer speech to inner speech involves truncation; the subtraction of context; and the omission of the subject of the sentence (the person speaking) but preservation of its predicate (the combination of action with place or object). I have proposed (Cromby, 2007) that this process of abstraction and generalisation can be extended to include a further stage where inner speech falls entirely away, leaving behind its corresponding feelings. Whereas in the Vygotskian schema 'I must get away' becomes 'get away' or 'away',[5] even this single word can be silenced, leaving just the felt imperative to escape.

Before proceeding, some caveats are necessary. First, actual experience is diachronic rather than sequential: the speech of others can also 'complete' our own feelings, and the experience seized upon by inner speech always already includes feelings (and associated fragments of inner speech) constitutive of the moment immediately preceding. Second, feelings also get 'seized upon' by other feelings: for example, my feeling unable to concentrate on any single task because there are so many to complete can generate anxiety that further compounds my difficulties.[6] Third, sensuous corporeal practices can also seize upon feelings: a soothing gesture may do more in a single instant to resolve feelings of sadness than any amount of reasoning. Fourth, feelings already bear their own tendencies towards meaning – valences, intensities, textures – with which discursive meanings typically get aligned. And fifth, images and other sensory stimuli can also both complete and provoke feeling.

With these caveats in mind, it seems possible that it is through such an extension of the Vygotskian schema that many feelings of knowing are actually produced.[7] Two processes may be involved, in combination. The first, in Vygotskian fashion, is a process of abstraction and generalisation. The second, developing a proposal from Langer, involves the projection of feeling into symbolic (linguistic) activity, such that its elements come to 'embody' particular qualities. Projection, here, is not meant in the Freudian sense of a defence mechanism keeping difficult feelings out of awareness. It has the more immediately literal meaning that, in perception, feelings get projected onto the world, rather as a cinema projector displays images upon a screen. Just as in the cinema what we see is not the screen per se but the screen-with-image, so in perception generally we see a world already infused with feeling. Langer proposes that humans have a unique capacity to 'see' or objectify feeling in objects and symbols, both natural and created, and it is this capacity that feelings of knowing represent. This objectification

> lets the subjective element come back as an impingement and be perceived as an external datum, i.e. as a quality belonging to an independently existing object; and that object, which thus presents our own sensory feeling to us, is a primitive symbol...The very existence of 'things' is modelled on his inward expectation of strains, directions, and limitations of his felt actions.
>
> (Langer, 1982, p. 48)

On the one hand, then, words and phrases not universally relevant get stripped away. On the other, 'little' words like 'and' or 'but' get associated with these feelings of strain, direction and limitation. Together, these two processes render certain feelings (which, as Johnson suggests, might include those enabled by the sensori-motor cortex) meaningful within somatic ensembles that words helped arrange but which no longer depend entirely upon language for their conceptual meaning. This is adaptive because the removal of denotative representational content, and its replacement by a more generic sensuous abstraction, allows sense to be readily transferred across contexts, conferring the widest generality and range of convenience.

Ratner (2000) draws on sources including Vygotsky and Dewey to make a related argument with respect to emotional feelings, presenting copious examples demonstrating how cultural presumptions, economic arrangements and stratifications of social relations differentiate and nuance what are, for the most part, quite general biological capacities, in the process producing regimes of emotion reflective of cultural norms, modes of labour and reproduction, and associated power and gender relations. He shows, for example, how gendered differences in emotionality mirror men's and women's differentially stereotyped roles within the separate spheres of paid work and domesticity; and how, although previously it had been considered a character flaw, US women's envy was encouraged after the First World War to stimulate commodity sales and boost the economy.

Whilst Ratner's analysis is valuable, it has two potentially problematic aspects. First, he argues that

> the cultural-psychological analysis I have presented requires that biological mechanisms contribute little, if anything to the specific characteristics of emotion. Emotions are not physically independent of biological processes, since they require a physical medium... However, emotions are functionally autonomous.
>
> (Ratner, 2000, p. 25)

This is troublesome because Ratner not only concedes that some coarse tendencies towards feeling must be present at birth, but also acknowledges that "some transcultural similarity in emotions is undeniable" (op. cit., p. 17) and that "[w]hile cultural variations in emotional expression are critically important features of emotions, certain common expressions may also exist" (op. cit., p. 19). Hence, the evidence he presents in support of cultural and socio-economic determination simultaneously reveals consistencies and commonalities between cultures and across epochs. Evidence that shame differs between ancient Taoists and modern Koreans highlights the persistence, across many centuries, of bodily potentials for something recognisable as shame; evidence that feudal love differs from American colonial love and contemporary romantic love simultaneously shows how the capacity to enact what we call love traverses time and place; and evidence that the incidence of guilt in sub-Saharan Africans has increased with the spread of Protestant religious belief and its emphasis on personal responsibility nevertheless reveals shared, latent potentials to feel something that, in English, gets called 'guilt'.[8]

The second problem with Ratner's analysis is the considerable weight he places upon cultural concepts conceived in predominantly cognitive terms, as he claims that

> [c]oncepts not only determine whether or not particular emotions will occur, they also determine the nuanced, modulated quality of an emotion. Happiness, for instance, is quite different according to whether one is marveling at a sunset in the desert, solving a difficult problem that advances a field of knowledge, or watching a favorite team win a frenzied athletic contest in the final moments. The enjoyment in each case is modulated by complex concepts about nature,

self-pride, intelligence, science, fame, the social good, identifying with athletic teams, competitive struggle and victory.

(Ratner, 2000, p. 11)

There is here a covert image of the rational appraiser cognitively wielding formal concepts which then shape feeling. However, we do not have to imagine that individuals typically wield concepts in this conscious manner in order to understand how culture and language nuance and differentiate emotional feeling. Indeed, what Ratner describes as cultural concepts are perhaps better understood as normative assumptions un-reflexively carried within linguistic and – especially – corporeal practices. Such practices are massively varied, sharing only their medium which is the physical body and the ways its sensorium and capacities can be entrained and educated through touch, sight, sound, comportment, gesture and movement. Whilst corporeal practices might frequently be enacted within dialogues, albeit dialogues very often seemingly about other things, their modality is therefore physical, sensual, gestural, imitative and physiognomic. Consequently, corporeal practices are able to engage whatever biologically endowed coarse tendencies towards emotional feeling that we may have long before the concepts Ratner implicates. In the initial enculturation of emotional feeling these practices therefore seem likely to predominate over, and be efficacious before, linguistic practices capable of carrying the relatively elaborate concepts Ratner implicates. Cultural norms nevertheless permeate and structure these corporeal practices, regulating them by being presumed within them, just as they simultaneously presume coarse bodily capacities that, by means of such presumption, get differentiated and stabilised as precisely the emotions proper to *that* culture, epoch and social position, rather than to any other.

These corporeal practices might be conceptualised with respect to the embodied aspects of the relational patterns of emotion described by Burkitt (2014). They might also be understood with respect to the somatic repertoires that bodily reproduce SES and gender distinctions, and that nuance these with more proximal influences conveyed, for example, through employment. Simultaneously, as a subsequent section of this chapter will suggest, we can also conceptualise these practices in relation to disciplinary regimes that create docile bodies by instilling normative subjectivities. In each case, their acquisition seems likely to elude conscious reflection and deliberate choice, and to be bound up with the acquisition of habits: of speaking, of thinking, of feeling, of sensing, of moving, holding and relating to the body. Although these various corporeal practices are often organised by (and run within) corresponding discursive practices they are not self-identical with these.[9] Their separate identification is necessary because their effects upon feeling are largely un-mediated by representation, making them harder to resist or reflect upon.

Notwithstanding these two problems, Ratner's account of the differentiation of emotional feeling is both insightful and supported by extensive evidence. Ratner also briefly addresses extra-emotional feelings of pain and sexual arousal. He describes evidence that feelings of pain (as measured both by pain thresholds and tolerance levels) are variable even though the physiological mechanisms sub-serving them are universal, and likewise that sexual arousal measured by physiological engorgement of the vaginal walls does not necessarily correlate with women's reported levels of arousal. His analysis nevertheless implicitly concurs with the suggestion from Chapter 3 that, relatively, these feelings are more socialised than socially or culturally differentiated. Considered more broadly, his analysis is also valuable because it emphasises how:

all thinking entails feelings e.g., thinking about going to work entails feelings of displeasure while thinking about going home entails pleasurable feelings; thinking about a problem entails feelings of frustration, despair, or excitement. Similarly, all feelings entail thinking – I'm sad about going to work because of how I remember work was recently and expect it to be today. Artistic work which is regarded as emotion-laden and emotion-driven is not purely emotional; it requires serious cognitive planning and reflection. Conversely, scientists are not devoid of emotions in their work. They are passionate about their work, they feel a sense of intrigue, frustration, satisfaction, and even elation and aesthetic appreciation at discovering a new phenomenon or formulating an elegant theory.

(Ratner, 2000, p. 6)

Thus, whilst it might sometimes seem that inner speech can operate independently of feeling, it is more accurate to recognise that inner speech is actually over-determined by feeling.[10] As we deliberate, the 'little' words that carry and direct reasoning – the if's, but's, and's, why's – are freighted, in the moments of their enactment, with felt senses of possibility, obstruction, connection and uncertainty. Likewise, the phrases that carry the meanings we reason about get produced in the unspoken equivalent of tones of voice that are emphatic, querulous, excited, despondent, impatient, measured, despairing, confident, bored, hopeful and so on. Inner speech is always subject to spontaneous excitation and felt provocation, and is both embodied and felt: its process is accompanied by motor activation of the musculature that produces ordinary speech (Locke & Fehr, 1970), and inhibiting this (by requiring people to clamp their mouths shut) can inhibit reasoning (Sokolov, 1975).

Simultaneously, frequently used words and phrases may have been intertwined with so many different feelings that they now seem largely devoid of felt significance: their mobilisation simply feels smooth, effortless and automatic. It is easy to mistake these subtle feelings of ease for an absence of feeling, and a short leap from there to imagine the existence of an independent faculty of cognition, a kind of "constant, standard competence" akin to a computer circuit (Langer, 1967, p. 149). This tendency can be further amplified by the metaphorical and homophonic connections these words and phrases may have with others, connections which – by illuminating possible directions in thinking – may also reinforce the illusion of a separable capacity of cognition. This illusion is further bolstered by cultural tendencies to sharply divide reason from feeling and, amongst psychologists, by the prominence of information-processing metaphors which are so ubiquitous that their metaphorical status is all but forgotten. In actuality, however:

> symbolic activity begets its own data for constant interpretation and reinterpretation, and its characteristic feelings, especially of strain and expectation, vagueness and clearness, ease and frustration, and the very interesting 'sense of rightness' that closes a finished thought process, as it guarantees any distinct intuition.[11]
>
> (Langer, 1967, p. 147)

## Felt experience

Although feelings are already both socialised and embodied, their intimate quality can make them seem the most private elements of experience and mislead scholars into imagining they can be studied as largely individual phenomena. For example, Johnson's (2007) otherwise insightful analysis of feelings of knowing suggests that these feelings might be enabled by the sensori-motor cortex: that bodily capacities to push, pull, resist, balance and so on provide the embodied, neural bases of felt reasoning processes. Whilst this proposal is enticing, Johnson's account does not adequately consider the contribution of socio-cultural resources, practices, structures and relations to the embodied meaning-making it describes. There are discussions of Stern's work on infant–parent interaction, of social insects, of traditions of food washing amongst Japanese macaque monkeys and of the language abilities of chimps; but there is no sustained consideration of work such as Vygotsky's that specifically considers *human* reasoning, and which treats it as already social in just the same way that Johnson treats it as already embodied.

Johnson acknowledges this omission, stating that "a fully adequate treatment of the social and cultural dimensions of thought would require substantially more evidence and analysis" (p. 151). However, he does not acknowledge that without this evidence and analysis, it is impossible to understand how we might sensibly have one feeling rather than another, or to explain how the 'correct' feeling might ever arise. He talks about feelings such as 'and' or 'but' – as Langer talks about feelings of ease, frustration, clarity and expectation – but these feelings seem to arise independently of learning or education, as though by some mysterious process the body already 'knows' how to feel. This makes it impossible for Johnson to adequately explain how someone might come to appropriately feel 'but' – as opposed to say 'and' – in response to a particular claim.

The recognition that feelings of knowing are constituted by association, both with prior inner speech (itself derived, through outer speech, from previous social interaction) and with previous corporeal practice, renders their meaningful character explicable. We appropriately feel 'but' – rather than 'and' – because our history of engagement with the topic, of reading and listening to similar arguments, our education in this and other fields, our upbringing and enculturation, acquisition of language and our experience of its interpenetration of and by sensual practice in the material world, jointly endow us with the capacity to sensibly mobilise those feelings as elements within a broader sensory gestalt. Johnson's suggestion that the sensori-motor cortex *enables* (some of) these feelings might be correct, but this does not mean it spontaneously causes them (Harre, 2002).

At the same time, because these are a-representational *feelings*, the sense they bear can shape experience in ways we might sometimes retrospectively recognise, but at the time might struggle to even notice. Their operation can therefore introduce a kind of patterned irrationality into thinking and relating. This is not to claim that feeling per se is irrational: feeling is integral to all reasoning and thinking. Rather, socially derived feelings of knowing can impel thoughts and relational choices broadly consistent with aspects of past experience, but somewhat disjunctive with – and occasionally maladaptive within – present circumstances. Recall that, like Johnson (2007), Billig's account of Freudian repression highlighted the significance of 'little' words and phrases like 'oh well' and 'but'. However, Billig did not theorise the felt element of these or other linguistic terms, rendering his analysis somewhat disembodied. The understanding that these 'little' words and phrases are already enactments of feeling, and that they bear a sense derived from prior social relations, begins to redress this absence.

In this regard, Langer's analysis of feelings has interesting parallels with Billig's work. As Chapter 2 explained, she recognises that a great many feelings are never symbolised or made objects of representation, and that "all conscious experience is symbolically conceived experience; otherwise it passes unrealised" (Langer, 1967, p. 100). Hence, just as Billig demonstrates that relational processes mediated by language can direct repression, Langer recognises that it is necessary to represent feelings for their full significance to be recognised. Likewise, Billig shows how repression is learned in conversation and interaction, whilst Langer emphasises that what is not discussed will likely be forgotten. So both Langer and Billig recognise that language plays a part in repression, with Billig identifying its relational origins and Langer conceptualising the feelings with which it works.

Langer's work might therefore allow Billig's relational analysis of repression to be more thoroughly situated within embodied, material contexts of relating. Feeling is a phase of the body, and the body is always spatio-temporally engaged with the world: consequently, we are "overburdened... not only with excessive sensibility, but also too many emotive impulses, certainly more than can be freely, overtly spent, especially in the social context of human life" (Langer, 1972, p. 277). As we move through the world, our bodies generate many more impulses towards feeling than we can enact and represent. The flux of ordinary activity, enabled by continuous bodily processes, inevitably produces more feelings than can be seized upon: there is simply not time to represent them all.

Whilst Langer said little about Freudian psychoanalysis, the production of this inevitable excess seems to be amongst the considerations that led her to describe the Freudian unconscious as a reification and its theoretical basis as 'over-assumptive' (Langer, 1967, p. 23). For her, the relational processes that Billig describes operate within a wider material frame of necessary excess, of interpellated feelings that – for wholly contingent reasons impelled by spatio-temporal actualities largely external to the subject – nevertheless evade linguistic completion. The Freudian unconscious reifies complex, interweaving sets of material and relational processes, misrepresenting their combined effects as personal dynamics wholly impelled by hidden sources – drives – buried within the individual. This obscures how embodied experience within a material world constantly stimulates excesses of feeling that cannot all be seized upon, and how – within this melee – there is nevertheless a circumscribed role for the interpersonal dynamics of repression that Freud described and Billig explains.

It is important to emphasise that these interpersonal dynamics are always both relational and societal: they do not just reflect the personal sensitivities of taboos, shame, embarrassment, guilt and anxiety, they also – simultaneously – reflect wider societal forces, institutions and concerns. Billig (1999, pp. 220–252) provides an excellent illustration of this, in his reading of Freud's account of his conversation with Dora about her experience of spending two hours being transfixed by Raphael's *Madonna* and yet, seemingly, being unable to account for its fascination. Billig first observes that Freud does not seem especially interested in this unusual experience, relegating his (for Billig, unconvincing) interpretation to a footnote. He also observes that Freud's interpretation demonstrates how his analysis of Dora consistently emphasised interpersonal, relational, sexual and presumed intra-psychic processes. In so doing, Billig suggests, Freud's interpretation colludes with Dora's own seeming inability to explain, because both sidestep the most compellingly obvious explanation: the likely anxiety produced for both of them by the virulent and rising anti-Semitism of the time.

### Radical individuality

So whether we emphasise inner speech or whether we emphasise feeling, we see that individual felt experience is also simultaneously social. But this does not mean that individuality is illusory, that individuals are not unique or are somehow determined by social forces. Rather, it suggests a kind of radical individuality to experience. No two people ever have quite 'the same' experience of anything, because everyone brings to each moment a unique trailing history of prior moments, a specific trajectory of being forged from particular contingent combinations of biology, culture, materiality and sociality. Consequently, every generalisation cuts across these unique experiences in ways that sometimes illuminate and sometimes obscure. From this perspective, individual experience is radical because it *necessarily* exceeds the psychological laws said to regulate it.

At the same time, individual experience is radical because it is largely composed of elements common to all. It is enabled by elements of the same flesh, with similar capacities for feeling, movement, reaction and appraisal; mediated by similar material organisations of tools, artefacts, resources, situations, locations and institutions; organised by shared narratives, discourses and practices; regulated by enduring constellations of distal powers that distribute uneven concentrations of resources, both material and cultural; and realised and reflected upon in accord with collectively held precepts that instantiate the boundaries, rights and obligations of selfhood. The radical individuality of experience resides, not in the elements of which it is forged, but in the dynamic, historically, culturally and biologically contingent conjunctions by which it gets constituted.

## Subjectivity and habit

A notion of habit is already implicated within Vygotsky's account of the acquisition of inner speech, which depends upon repetitions that produce the capacities for abstraction and generalisation that render certain words and phrases as habitual. To this extent, we can already see how habit, "understood as a form of more-or-less automated repetition" (Bennett et al., 2013, pp. 4–5), shapes and co-constitutes experience. Moreover, because all experience occurs in material settings shaped by specific power relations and associated configurations of roles, resources, spaces and places, habit can embed the consequences of power within experience by aligning it with distinct, disciplined modes of experience: subjectivities.[12] Foucault's work, which emphasised the connections between disciplinary power and disciplined, compliant subjectivities, encourages the association of habit with the 'docile bodies' he described. As Bennett et al. (2013, p. 3) say, "habit has typically constituted a point of leverage for regulatory practices that seek to effect some realignment of the relations between different components of personhood". More generally, psychology identifies habitual feelings, typically associated with exposure to noxious situations, in relation to concepts such as low self-esteem (Brown, 1993) and stigma (Dinos et al., 2004). Moreover, many mental health problems can be understood as being constituted, to a significant extent, of habitual feelings derived from unpleasant experiences of various kinds (Romme et al., 2009).

Nevertheless, habit is not solely a conduit for unreflexive activity that aligns with power relations and reproduces dominant forms of subjectivity: habit also frees us from needing to monitor activity too closely, generating capacities for deliberation and choice. Following Dewey, Bennett et al. (2013, p. 12) observe that habits can be understood as "parts of mind-body-environmental assemblages" or "things done by the environment by means of organic structures or acquired dispositions". Habits are relays between the material and social world and the realm of experience that operate by structuring and organising the capacities of the body. Consequently, habits can help as well as hinder; they can generate compliance as well as facilitate subversion: but all these capacities flow from both their automaticity and their responsiveness.

Merleau-Ponty (2002, p. 175) similarly argued that because habits organise the body, including its sensations and its actions, they also condition perception: "every habit is both motor and perceptual, because it lies, as we have said, between explicit perception and actual movement, in the basic function which sets boundaries to our field of vision and our field of action." Experience is pre-reflectively finessed by habitually enacted regimes of movement and perception: Harre (1999) writes of learning how to 'grade' sheep fleeces for quality by recognising minute differences of look and feel that would be invisible to those without practice; wine connoisseurs learn to make increasingly fine-graded judgements regarding the tastes, scents and colours associated with grapes, regions and vintages; likewise, music producers train their hearing, through repeated listening, such that they eventually discern resonances and interferences others cannot (Cox, 2014). Again, habit does not only constrain, and repetition does not only induce dull mechanical uniformities (although, as everyone who has been employed will affirm, this it surely can do). In appropriate circumstances, if its affordances are cultivated and subtle gradations of difference in repetition recognised and reflexively considered, habit educates perception to reveal degrees of difference that were previously imperceptible.

The primary context for analyses of habit that highlight its potentials to both instil conformity and facilitate reflection is provided by readings of Foucault's work which imply that regimes of discourse seemingly drill their effects down to the very smallest level, imposing subjectivities uniformly aligned with disciplinary requirements. This means that everyday practices of resistance, subversion, non-compliance, paying lip service or being ironically overenthusiastic cannot be explained. Subjectification – deliberate work upon the self in order to be a particular kind of person pursuing a specific project – gets wholly aligned with subjection (to all-encompassing regimes of power), ultimately making it impossible to imagine how social change or political trans-formation could ever occur. Hence, contemporary analyses of habit highlight its liberatory potentials alongside its constraining tendencies, emphasising the capacities for reflection and enhanced perception it affords whilst recognising how it constrains and regulates. Reference has already been made to the post-Foucauldian notion of 'continous experi-ence' developed by Stephenson and Papadopoulos (2007), within which the limitations, gaps and contradictions of dominant discourses con-tinuously create eruptions of discord and uncertainty that may foment alternate understandings and subversive alignments. Experience there-fore always potentially exceeds the discursive regimes that regulate it, and these excesses generate possibilities for wider social change. Notions of excess are also highlighted within political analyses that emphasise how experiences of protest and resistance offer fleeting, intense glimpses of alternative social orders and their corresponding ways of being and relating (The Free Association, 2011).

It nevertheless remains necessary to emphasise that power does consistently operate by regulating the discourses and practices driv-ing the habits that form subjectivities, and to realise that this can happen quite subtly. There is, for example, a paradox in Langer's anal-ysis of the relationship between art and feeling that, perhaps, reflects her own privileged circumstances. Langer endows art with the capac-ity to both objectify feeling and re-fashion subsequent experience by acting back upon ways of perceiving. Whilst this analysis explic-itly includes literature, she does not grant similar powers to everyday language, even though it also contributes to the constitution of experi-ence. Some years ago the fictional biography of a computer-generated meerkat from a television advertisement was a UK bestseller (Orlov, 2010). This instance of the penetration of everyday experience by cul-turally proffered tokens has been analysed from the perspectives of marketing studies (Patterson, Khogeer, & Hodgson, 2012) and ideol-ogy critique (Khalliatt, 2013). Yet the appeal of studies demonstrating how such cultural forms can be taken up ironically, archly or sub-versively sometimes obscures the extent to which they are also used uncritically, unthinkingly, even unknowingly. Many people frequently interpret their experience through the tropes, discourses and narra-tives of advertising, popular music, Hollywood films, celebrity gossip and television soap operas, just as others from different backgrounds routinely invoke art-house cinema, classic literature or Shakespearean theatre – simply because this is what they are most frequently exposed to, and what is presented as already normative.[13] Neither their banality, nor the profound ways they open up experience to ideology and power, negate how these *everyday* elements are as thoroughly constitutive of experience as those we venerate as art.

## Conclusion

Language and feeling are not the whole of experience. However, they are amongst its most prominent elements, and their influence is all but continuous. Placing feeling at the root of experience, and conceptualising feeling as an emergent phase of the living body, grounds experience in the material and social world. Simultaneously, situating experience on the mobile, slippery boundary between 'inner' and 'outer' – between what is felt as endogenous and what is felt as exogenous, and between what is merely felt and what is both felt and completed by language – enables its socially and relationally driven complexities to be considered equally alongside its embodied aspects. From this perspective, we might ultimately begin to understand how a great many psychological phenomena – not just emotions, but also dreams, fantasies, wishes, desires, beliefs, attitudes, opinions – are co-constituted in and through experiential dynamics that centrally include feeling and language.

# 5
# Researching

In the first volume of *Mind*, Langer reproduces an assessment of the nature and quality of psychological research, taken from a 1959 work by Sigmund Koch (where, in turn, Koch attributes it to an earlier conversation with Charles Tolman):

> [T]o me, the journals seem to be full of over-sophisticated mathematical treatments of data which are in themselves of little intrinsic interest and of silly little findings which, by a high powered statistic, can be proved to contradict the null hypothesis.
>
> (cited in Langer, 1967, p. 51)

In the decades since Tolman expressed this opinion, the primary focus of psychological research has changed. Before 1959 the dominant paradigm was behaviour; by 1967 cognition had mostly taken its place; today, neuroscience and the brain are increasingly influential. Research has also become considerably more sophisticated, largely due to the ready availability (in many parts of the world) of various new technologies: powerful computers with sophisticated software to run experiments, manage data and conduct analyses; behavioural recording devices such as actimeters; and high-quality, portable audio and video recorders. These technologies have facilitated new methods and designs, allowing psychologists to record and analyse considerably more complexity and detail than before.

Notwithstanding the successive dominance of different overarching paradigms, psychology remains relatively diverse. These paradigms were never entirely homogenous: cognitive psychology, for example, accommodates a variety of substantive foci, theories and methods. Simultaneously, other theories – psychodynamic, poststructuralist, constructionist, systemic, humanist – have had an enduring influence, alongside concepts drawn from medical, clinical, forensic, organisational and educational fields. Consequently, the fault lines that fragment psychology into sub-disciplines reflecting wider dualistic assumptions sometimes facilitate substantive and methodological diversity. Within social psychology, for example, the discursive paradigm is an important model of cognition that challenges the isolated monads of mainstream psychology by demonstrating how thinking is as much joint, public and discursive as individual, private and computational. Diversity is apparent with respect to methods, with increased recognition of the value of qualitative, pluralistic and mixed methods research, in social psychology and in the discipline more generally. In the UK, the British Psychological Society now mandates qualitative methods teaching as an element of all accredited psychology undergraduate degrees, and the American Psychological Association recently inaugurated a Society for Qualitative Inquiry (Division 5) and an associated journal (*Qualitative Psychology*).

It is tempting to interpret these developments as elements of a singular narrative of progress. However, psychology's situation and character – straddling the biological and socio-cultural, primarily oriented towards practical applications and empirical findings, and for these and other reasons prone to recurrent crises (Parker, 1989) – suggests this would be an over-simplification. Although effect sizes are now more frequently reported, research remains very largely dependent upon notions of statistical – as opposed to, say, clinical – significance (Jacobson & Truax, 1991), and many critics argue that journals are *still* mostly filled with studies that, whilst mathematically sophisticated, have little intrinsic interest or wider import (Fox, Prilletensky, & Austin, 2009; Moloney, 2013).

If psychology were nevertheless accumulating a substantial stock of valid knowledge, some over-production of trivial findings as epiphenomenon would be reasonable. However, Simmons, Nelson and Simonsohn (2011) found that psychology researchers routinely exploit flexibility in the conduct and reporting of statistical analysis in order to dramatically inflate the apparent rate of positive findings. Pashler and Wagenmakers (2012) describe a "crisis in confidence" engendered by a number of high-profile fraud cases; the publication in a high-profile journal of experimental evidence for extra-sensory perception; reports that psychologists are frequently unwilling to share data for re-analysis by colleagues; a widespread reluctance to even attempt replication; and high-profile failures to replicate some findings. Likewise, Kühberger,

Fritz and Scherndl (2014) meta-analysed effect sizes in a random sample of nearly 400 papers and demonstrated a strong publication bias across psychology, typically achieved by reporting unexpected significances as though they had always been the study goal.

So far at least, these graphic demonstrations of how quantitative psychology is already distorted by interest have not engendered any widespread fundamental questioning of the extent to which a science of the human – in the natural scientific sense – is actually possible. Rather, disciplinary dynamics of power and interest (themselves enmeshed within larger circuits of monitoring, incentivisation and regulation – Lorenz, 2012) continue to produce a contradictory actuality within which quantitative research is still sometimes presented as *necessarily* more valuable than qualitative. Despite acknowledging that roughly half of UK social psychologists conduct qualitative research, a 2011 international benchmarking review jointly authored by the ESRC, British Psychological Society, Association of Heads of Psychology Departments and the Experimental Psychology Society asserted that "UK social psychology's international impact is almost exclusively attributable to its mainstream experimental/quantitative work". This unsupported claim was rapidly rebutted, using citation information to establish the significant international impact of UK qualitative social psychology (Billig et al., 2011). Nevertheless, both its blithe assertion, and the somewhat ironic need to use citation indices to challenge it, illustrates how a unitary narrative of progress is untenable. Psychological research is continuously contested, both internally and externally, and these ongoing contestations are shaping its evolving character.

It is not the aim of this chapter to provide a 'how to' guide for researchers, not least because there are excellent books of this kind already available. Instead, the chapter addresses the more modest aim of identifying some general difficulties and dilemmas attendant upon the empirical study of feeling in psychology. After a brief summary of some challenges that are frequently encountered, discussion will focus first upon quantitative methods, and then qualitative methods.

## Challenges

Whichever method is used, empirical studies of feeling are challenging because they necessarily rely upon data or measures – behavioural indices, questionnaires, interviews, photographs, observations of naturally occurring activities – that only imperfectly represent the ineffable, felt experience being studied. Whilst these challenges frequently apply to studies of other psychological phenomena, they may acquire particular force in relation to feeling because of its particular combination of intrinsic characteristics. Feeling is constitutive of experience, it is a-representational, and it is always bound up with people, places, situations and activities. Its full meaning is therefore realised only within the situated particularity of specific embodied moments – acts – of which representational data are at best only one aspect.

Sometimes the pervasiveness of these difficulties is largely disguised. For example, the various items on the Clinical Anger Scale (CAS) – (Snell et al., 1995) link feelings of anger to other feelings (hostility, tiredness, sexual desire) and to multiple activities (relating to others, sleeping, making love):

*Table 5.1*  Sample items from the Clinical Anger Scale (Snell et al., 1995)

| | |
|---|---|
| 1 | A. I do not feel angry. |
| | B. I feel angry. |
| | C. I am angry most of the time now. |
| | D. I am so angry and hostile all the time that I can't stand it. |
| 11 | A. Things are not more irritating to me now than usual. |
| | B. I feel slightly more irritated now than usual. |
| | C. I feel irritated a good deal of the time. |
| | D. I'm irritated all the time now. |
| 16 | A. My anger does not interfere with my sleep. |
| | B. Sometimes I don't sleep very well because I'm feeling angry. |
| | C. My anger is so great that I stay awake 1–2 hours later than usual. |
| | D. I am so intensely angry that I can't get much sleep during the night. |
| 21 | A. I don't feel so angry that it interferes with my interest in sex. |
| | B. My feelings of anger leave me less interested in sex than I used to be. |
| | C. My current feelings of anger undermine my interest in sex. |
| | D. I'm so angry about my life that I've completely lost interest in sex. |

The description of the CAS as an objective, valid self-report measure, it's use of four-point rating scales, and its compliance with statistical thresholds for internal consistency, validity, and reliability, nevertheless obscure how – because feeling is constitutive, a-representational, ineffable – the numbers it produces *cannot* be quantifying anger in any precise or straightforward sense.[1] But these characteristics of feeling also pose a challenge to qualitative researchers: firstly because large proportions of qualitative data consist of self-reports (collected in interviews, focus groups or diaries); secondly, because self-reports – and the great majority of qualitative data generally – are also linguistic.

Feeling is continuously interpellated by language, social relations, activity and situation. The dynamic processes of the feeling body are always inflected by nuances and impingements arising from attempts to achieve a goal, progress a relationship, satisfy a need, comfort a loved one and so on. Simultaneously, how we feel also reflects organismic dynamics, some of which depend upon circadian rhythms that regulate appetite and arousal in ways simultaneously both environmentally responsive and biologically organised (Roenneberg et al., 2007). Consequently, some days, we might feel 'foggy headed', stupefied or dulled, whereas on others we might feel refreshed, confident and enthusiastic, yet in both cases we might identify no sensible social, relational or environmental reason for this. Feeling is therefore contingent upon our biological constitution and its processes; upon the situations and relations we find ourselves within; and upon how these mobile, dynamic contingencies happen to intersect.

The challenge this poses for psychological research into feeling is that the great majority of studies depend upon particular set-ups (experiments, laboratories) measures (questionnaires, checklists) or procedures (interviews, diary entries, focus groups). If only because of the need for informed consent, there is almost no research which does not involve some deformation of, or intrusion into, the relational and embodied flows that would otherwise have occurred. Coupled with the frequent necessity to depend upon self-reports, this creates the continuous possibility that data are partial, incomplete and inflected with other considerations. Self-reported feelings of wellbeing, for example, are frequently influenced by social desirability (Cromby, 2011). Conversely, Scheff (2003) found that self-reports of shame were extremely rare, even when explicitly requested; he surmised that this is because shame feelings are so toxic that few participants were comfortable disclosing them.

These challenges flow directly from the analyses presented in the preceding chapters. In relation to quantitative method, they take on a particular cast because quantification necessarily imposes categories and boundaries upon what in actuality are seamlessly ongoing flows of experience. In relation to qualitative method, by contrast, the sharpest issues probably arise from the status of language and its relationship with feeling.

## Quantitative method

Danziger (1994) shows how psychology's disciplinary imperative towards quantification reflects historical attempts to make the discipline relevant by providing data about psychological constructs such as intelligence, personality and self-esteem. Since these constructs were thought to mediate the effects of policies and interventions, the consequent need to render them calculable created a niche within which psychology could develop. This established reciprocal relations of mutual regulation between psychology's methods and the problems it addressed. Having developed procedures to address one problem, expertise could be transferred to others – but only insofar as these were similar problems, amenable to similar kinds of investigation. Psychology's focus upon the individual meant that the problems it addressed were often related to practices of grading and social control (Michell, 2000). Intelligence tests, for example, sort students according to their apparent ability to think and learn, thus regulating their educational opportunities and life chances; personality tests are used in similar ways in occupational contexts, where they regulate access to employment.

Other influences also encouraged the rapid rise of quantitative method. Jones and Elcock (2001) identify personal and institutional imperatives to break from existing traditions of philosophical enquiry and develop an apparently natural science of human behaviour (impelled in part by Darwin's work), and show how the British statistical tradition (with its debt to hereditarian theories) was influential. Psychoanalysis also had a continuous if somewhat covert influence (Parker, 1997), as did the various broader social and technological changes associated with the rise of capitalism (Tolman, 1994) and the evolution of the modern state (Rose, 1985).

Nevertheless, it seems fair to conclude, with Danziger (1994), that it was within the everyday conduct of the very practical activities of responding to demands for a psychology that was applicable, relevant and marketable that these influences had their effects, and it was through their confluence within these activities that quantitative method quickly came to dominate psychology. This dominance is now largely taken for granted, and the practice of psychometrics – the measurement of mental capacities and operations – seen as largely routine. Studies frequently deploy psychometric measures of purportedly purely cognitive constructs, such as working memory and reasoning; of affectively inflected constructs such as attitudes, beliefs, self-esteem and self-efficacy; and of straightforwardly feeling-laden constructs such as wellbeing and emotion. Whilst researchers may expend considerable effort choosing appropriate measures for such constructs, they seem confident that measurement per se is both possible and appropriate.

It is surprising, then, that the foundational hypothesis of psychometrics – that psychological processes, states and capacities are actually amenable to quantification – seems never to have been tested. Michell (2000) shows that the quantification of psychological constructs involves two necessary tasks. The first 'scientific' task "involves devising test situations that are differentially sensitive to the presence or absence of quantitative structure" (op.cit., p. 649). The second 'instrumental' task involves creating valid measures that can reliably measure this attribute. We are only justified in attempting the second 'instrumental' task if the test situations deployed within the first 'scientific' task produced evidence that the attribute being investigated does have a quantitative character. For example, we are only justified in measuring anger using a rating scale if it has already been shown that anger varies in accord with the systematic intervals such scales presuppose.

Michell (2000) observes that whilst texts on psychometrics frequently present detailed expositions of multiple aspects of the instrumental task, they never engage with the scientific task that logically precedes this instrumental development. Snell et al. (1995) detail how they established the preliminary reliability and validity of the CAS by conducting factor analyses to establish its unidimensional structure, by calculating reliability coefficients and alphas to establish stability and internal consistency, and by correlating it with measures of related constructs (trait anger, state anger, anger control) in order to warrant validity. However, nowhere in this paper do they describe engaging with the scientific task of demonstrating that angry feelings are actually amenable to quantification.

Michel suggests that this peculiar situation came about largely because of the adoption of an 'anomalous' definition of measurement, coined by Stevens in 1946, as "the assignment of numerals to objects or events according to rule" (op.cit., p. 650). In combination with the uptake from physics of the procedure of operationism (where the meaning of a concept is understood as the set of operations that specify it) this concept of 'measurement as rule-generation' has allowed researchers to sidestep the need to validate measurement against the qualities of the attribute itself. Instead, psychometrics proceeds:

> by stipulating that the theoretical attribute is quantitative and that this attribute is quantitatively related to the relevant test scores. Since these issues are empirical, stipulation here substitutes for scientific investigation, a substitution disguised by the doctrine of operationism combined with Stevens' definition of measurement.
>
> (Michell, 2000, p. 657)

Feeling constitutes experience by ebbing, flowing, moving and changing. With the exception of unusual, abrupt intrusions (the sudden pain of, say, stubbing your toe) its textures and valences rarely arise discretely or episodically. Feeling might surge rapidly, it might build gradually, it might dissipate suddenly or linger for days, but in all these movements it does not seem to vary in discrete units that can be precisely enumerated. Langer (1967) was sceptical of the ability of language to represent feeling precisely because of this kind of problem (see Chapter 4). Yet, as the CAS illustrates, this is how measurement proceeds. An initial process of linguistic conversion uses words to (imprecisely) represent feeling; then either a tick box (yes/no), a check list or – as in the CAS – a rating scale format is used to transform these words into numbers. Whilst these processes of linguistic and numerical conversion are discrepant with the actual characteristics of feeling, they create the superficial appearance of precise measurement.

Demonstrating how this apparent precision is produced, Rosenbaum and Valsiner (2011) conducted a novel empirical study interrogating quantification using rating scales. They asked participants to respond to statements from the widely used NEO PI-R personality inventory, using a Likert scale ranging from 'false' to 'true' – but in a novel way. Before marking the scale, in relation to each statement participants had to first write what they took 'false' and 'true' to mean in relation to that item; then, after marking a scale point, to write a brief rationale for their answer. Over 100 participants, divided roughly equally between Estonia and the USA, completed this procedure for 14 statements from the NEO PI-R.

Analysis of this data showed that the meanings of 'false' and 'true' differed substantially, not only between participants, but also between questions. Far from simply introspecting and then reporting objectively the extent to which a given statement was true or false for them, participants first interpreted the statement then evaluated themselves in relation to their own interpretation. By 'slowing down' the usually rapid process of scale completion, Rosenbaum and Valsiner showed how the meanings of 'false' and 'true' were related in distinct 'dialogical fields' temporarily constructed in relation to each item. They used their findings to challenge the accepted belief that rating scales comprise a neutral, objective medium of psychological measurement, instead concluding that

> it is a misplaced assumption that participants have direct access to their response and that this response is static and can be represented as a mark along a line...rating scale data, despite being

statistically manipulated, should not (and indeed cannot) be thought of as objective.

(Rosenbaum & Valsiner, 2011, p. 61)

Whilst these analyses refer to quantification generally, they are clearly relevant to feeling. An apparent paradox nevertheless arises because, for the most part, participants faced with instruments such as the CAS do not hold up their hands in bewilderment. Feelings of anger might alternatively be described as feelings of fury, sullenness, aggression, impatience, discontent and so on. Simultaneously, such feelings are interpellated fluidly by situations, events, discourses and practices, their boundaries are mobile and indeterminate and their intensities and textures moving and changing. Instruments such as the CAS ignore much of this variability and complexity, bracketing off the changing influence of places, people and situations with which angry feelings are associated (Eatough & Smith, 2006). Nevertheless, participants presented with the four choices of the CAS items seem able to choose one: the CAS, in other words, has face validity. Moreover, their choices exhibit some degree of consistency over time: the CAS is also reliable.

Harre (2002) offers an explanation for this paradox that, in accounting for the reliability and validity of questionnaires such as the CAS, casts further doubt on their ability to conduct accurate measurement. He suggests that psychometric questionnaires actually model psychological processes, rather than measuring them, and that this modelling explains their apparent validity and reliability. Harre argues that, when psychology borrowed many of its early methods and ontological presuppositions from physics, it overlooked the important distinction physicists make between instruments and apparatus. Instruments are things like thermometers: devices that change their physical state under the causal influence of some changing property of the environment. Apparatus refers to devices that function as laboratory analogues of real-world systems: for example, a gas discharge tube is an apparatus that models the dynamics of the upper atmosphere of our planet, and its electrical current models the effects of the solar wind. Apparatus has many uses, such as generating predictions about the possible future states of real-world systems. However, it cannot be used for measurement: only instruments, whose momentary properties depend causally upon aspects of the changing environment, can be used this way.

Questionnaires, Harre observes, are not instruments in the manner of thermometers. When participants give written or spoken answers, mark a checklist or tick a rating scale, they are doing nothing other than answering (in particular, formalised ways) questions posed by a psychologist. Consequently, there is not a consistent causal relation between participants' (presumed) psychological states and their questionnaire responses. Anger does not exert a determinate force that always makes participants choose particular rating scale points on the CAS. There is not the law-like relation between anger and these points that exists between the volume of a quantity of mercury and its temperature. This is because what actually occurs is not a process of measurement, but a precisely arranged, carefully structured, pre-emptively coded linguistic interaction. The CAS and other psychometric questionnaires are analogues of everyday conversations: effectively, they are apparatus, not instruments. This means that whilst they can model psychological processes, they cannot sensibly be said to measure them. Regardless of the intentions of those who use them, and irrespective of the painstaking work that goes into their construction and testing, it is a conceptual error to interpret their outcomes as measurements.

It follows that neither the reliability nor the face validity of these questionnaires are a function of their ability to measure psychological processes. Instead, both are entirely explicable as by-products of the same shared, normative precepts that sustain everyday conversation. These precepts derive from two sources: the semantic rules for understanding the meaning of terms such as 'angry', and the autobiographical and narrative conventions that obtain when telling information to relative strangers in unusual situations. Because these rules and conventions are widely shared, self-report questions that invoke them can be readily answered (face validity). Similarly, consistency (reliability) in people's answers reflects their shared orientation to these cultural conventions and semantic rules, just as variation reflects the degrees of freedom these conventions bestow.

These difficulties are frequently compounded by others that flow from the way quantitative findings are typically produced by either summing or averaging the numbers that psychometric measures generate. Tolman (1994) observes how in most psychological research we first isolate the person, who is characteristically assessed alone (whilst Tolman's focus is the experiment, this holds largely true for other designs). The person's responses – already fragmentary, partial, tangential and static by comparison with their flowing, situated, embodied experience of, say, anger – are recorded as a numerical abstraction generated, for example, by the CAS. Typically, this number then gets summed or averaged with those abstracted from other participants, thus generating higher-level abstractions even further divorced from the radical individuality of each person's felt experience. The differences between group means in these abstractions are then compared with their associated variance, using statistics to estimate the likelihood of their arising by chance. The overall process is one of increasing distance from lived experience, of its particularities being substituted by abstract numbers with relatively tenuous relations to the phenomenal actualities they purportedly represent. Tolman (1994, p. 53–54) concludes that: "the actual movement is from the very concrete level of an individual human life to a level of abstraction at which no concrete individual existence is any longer recognizable".

A further challenge for quantitative studies is that how we feel now is simultaneously dependent upon how we felt in the moment just preceding, and upon what we are doing, where we are and who we are with. The inner speech we attach to feeling is also contingent upon prior moments, whilst also being open to normative influences aligned with dominant cultural understandings. These 'inner' dialectics are always dynamically interwoven with 'outer' dialectics, so that felt experience gets continuously reconstituted on the somewhat fluid boundary between self and others. Yet, because of its necessary dependence upon rigid categories imposed by psychometric instruments and other operationalised variables, quantitative method artificially constrains much of this dynamism. Whilst this (sometimes) allows it to produce statistically significant associations, at the same time it largely occludes any understanding of which *specific* associations will be most relevant in which particular circumstances.

These problems do not mean that quantitative measures of feeling are entirely without merit. To some extent they can be attenuated by experience sampling techniques such as the day reconstruction method (Kahneman et al., 2004): whilst these studies still rely upon self-reports, their temporal immediacy increases their capacity to meaningfully capture something of the changing textures of experience. Tolman (1994) suggests that the generalised knowledge produced by quantitative studies is of the kind that politicians, managers or bureaucrats might find useful in their efforts to influence or predict how people will think, act and feel. Ratner (2000) argues that quantitative method might be useful in relation to studies exploring broad-brush associations between social structures and emotional experiences. For example, Illousz (2012) argues that the psychologisation of workplace emotion was welcomed by workers because it democratised social relations. In order to establish whether this claim holds, or whether it was experienced primarily as an intensification of surveillance and control, some kind of quantitative enquiry seems necessary. Similarly, Harre (2002) argues that psychometric measures generate coarse indices of the subject positions typically taken up when people answer questions posed by psychologists (and others), and that knowledge of the broad patterns of these positions might be useful.

Counter-intuitively, then, quantitative psychological measures of feeling seem better at indexing abstract generality than contextualised specificity. But when applied to individual feeling they typically render the enmeshed social, relational and material processes that continuously constitute it as mere static background. The imaginary truth of felt experience is revealed by seemingly stripping away societal, relational and material influences; by synthetically constraining (but not removing) the social relations of the present moment; and by converting verbal traces of felt experience into quantities, in ways that superficially approximate to objective measurement. Together, these concerns constitute significant obstacles to the quantitative psychological study of felt experience.

Advocates of quantitative method might challenge this conclusion. They might counter that feeling can be readily assessed using appropriate study designs, participant selection and randomisation procedures, suitable modes and orders of stimulus presentation, apt response measures and appropriate analyses. These technical matters dominate research methods training, allowing psychologists to (nominally) address many relevant phenomena. It is nevertheless worth reflecting upon the sheer quantity of detailed considerations these procedures contain, the mass of research using and refining them, the status afforded this research and those proficient in its conduct, the considerable time and effort expended grasping its intricacies, perfecting its skills and practicing its styles of thought, and the cool yet sensuous pleasures, the feelings of mastery, that accompany their application. All this, and it is not surprising that some quantitative psychologists will inevitably *feel* that this conclusion is unreasonable.[2]

## Qualitative method

Wertz (2011) observes that qualitative data was important for such seminal figures as James, Freud, Erikson, Piaget, Kohlberg, Allport, Maslow and Rogers; that as long ago as 1894 Dilthey argued that the methods of psychology would always necessarily differ from those of the natural sciences in that they necessarily require some engagement with meaning; and that in 1942 Allport published a lengthy review of extant psychological research utilising autobiographies, interviews, diaries, letters and similar sources. Despite these historically important contributions, it is only in recent decades that qualitative methods have accounted for notable proportions of psychological research. Their impact has nevertheless been steadily increasing, and Willig and Stainton-Rogers (2007) describe how qualitative methods are increasingly supported by funding bodies, how recommendations for 'evidence based practice' in healthcare now incorporate qualitative evidence, and how editorial boards of major journals frequently include people with qualitative expertise. Qualitative psychological research today is characterised by innovation: the contributors to Reavey (2011) demonstrate the considerable potentials of visual methods, and there is increasing interest in analyses involving other participant-generated or supplied objects and images – maps, drawings, photographs, poems, songs, memorabilia and so on. Mixed methods studies combining qualitative and quantitative techniques continue to attract attention, and there is growing interest in the potentials of qualitative analytical pluralism (the use of two or more qualitative methods to analyse the same set of data – Clarke et al., 2015). These developments raise paradigmatic, ontological and epistemological questions which are also being addressed, for example using the concept of bricolage (Kincheloe & Berry, 2004).

At the same time, qualitative methods still encounter resistance. Danziger (1994) showed how quantitative method allowed psychology to align itself with powerful interests; similarly, Wertz (2011, p. 85) observes that "by employing research methods of natural science, university departments of psychology have built laboratories, funded graduate assistants, and won economic support". Many qualitative researchers have recognised and responded to this context by demonstrating their own capacities to generate useful psychological knowledge – although some misguidedly argue that it is actually the prominence of theory and diversity of methods in qualitative research that produces its subsidiary status. The proliferation of quality criteria for qualitative research (e.g. Parker, 2004; Tracy, 2010) is similarly driven by researchers' interests in persuading funders, journal editors and other gatekeepers that rigour can be transparently assessed. Whilst such criteria may help assure standards they are also associated with methodological purism, as opposed to the flexible deployment of rigorous analytics in ways best suited to research questions and data (Chamberlain, Cain, Sheridan, & Dupuis, 2011).

It is therefore important to acknowledge that, just like quantitative techniques, qualitative methods are also technologies of reduction that artificially cut partial, static excerpts from the swirling flux of experience. Many studies depend solely upon one-time 'drive-by inter-views', a practice that explores the richness of participants' experiences only in comparatively restrictive ways (Chamberlain, 2012). Interviews also have considerable potential to saturate data with analyst's concerns whilst, simultaneously, fostering the illusion that what they access is 'real' attitudes or experiences (Potter & Hepburn, 2005). It is also occasionally possible to discern quasi-romantic suggestions of an analytic process that seemingly reflects the totality of experience, of an indulgent process within which the researcher's 'journey' is of central significance, or of suggestions that merely 'giving voice' to participants will, of itself, transform what is known and done. So qualitative psychological research has its own potentials for omission and occlusion, and is sometimes inflected with a naïve humanism that limits its analytic capacity.

Nevertheless, in qualitative studies participants self-evidently do have considerably more freedom, even within a single interview, than in response to questionnaires where response variation and contextual nuance are *systematically* excluded or suppressed (Potter & Wetherell, 1987). Moreover, although qualitative research sometimes depends upon engineered situations – the interview, the focus group, the memory work group – these situations far more closely resemble everyday conversation than the questionnaires used in quantitative method; qualitative analyses typically also incorporate theories and evidence that address broader considerations. There are, besides, many qualitative studies that analyse naturally occurring data, gathered from situations and interactions that would have occurred anyway. Overall, then, the degrees of artifice and misdirection in qualitative research are fewer, and the capacity of analytic procedures to transcend them greater. In addition, it's recursive character means qualitative research is better able to incorporate reflexive considerations flowing not only from the researcher's preferences, important though they are, but also from "the social and intellectual unconscious embedded in the analytic tools and operations" (Johnson, Long, & White, 2000, p. 248). For these reasons, qualitative methods are considerably better able than quantitative to engage psychologically with the ways that feelings are always already embedded in dynamic, cultural and material contexts of sociality and relationality.

## Language, feeling and meaning

Despite the increasing diversity of the data collected in some studies, qualitative research remains highly dependent on language. Both the data and what researchers presume to be knowable from it – its epistemology – are almost exclusively linguistic. Qualitative analysis typically involves identifying and then 'reading the significance' of spoken or written patterns, repertoires, tropes, clichés, gaps, contradictions, connotations, absences or contradictions in order to ascertain meanings (Madill, Jordan, & Shirley, 2000) which are, variously, understood to be produced within narratives, organised in discourses, contingent upon the organisation of conversational turns, constituted in the patterning of themes, invoked homonymically by similes or metaphors and so on.

The dominance of language is such that, sometimes, untenable claims for its capacity and reach are made. For example, in arguing that narrative analysis is sufficient to encompass embodied experiences, Phoenix and Orr (2014, p. 101) claim that "Experience... is nothing more than an enactment of pre-given stories" and that "it is the stories already circulating within society... that enable sensory, documented, habitual and immersive pleasures to be experienced". This claim, that pleasure itself is a story rather than an embodied experience, substitutes language for the body and in so doing obscures the many ways in which combinations of sensory capacities, corporeal practices, embodied habits and arrangements of cultural and material resources enable pleasure to be both experienced and documented. It prioritises the retrospective narratives gathered in research over the immanent contingencies of the flow of lived experience wherein feeling and language constantly dialectically infuse each other. So to the extent that narratives of embodied pleasure do accurately capture the prior experiences to which they refer, their analysis does not obviate the need to *also* analyse feeling: just as it would make little sense to study the movements of a roller coaster without also considering the track upon which it runs. Nevertheless, in such ways, the feeling body is fleetingly acknowledged and then all too quickly marginalised. In these and other writings, the meaning of 'meaning' is commonly either taken to be self-evident, or is simply asserted as textual in accord with this dominant linguistic epistemology. Consequently, the ways that felt, bodily tendencies generate their own corporeal contributions to meaning that run alongside and within those of language are relatively rarely considered because as Braun and Clarke (2013, p. 1) acknowledge, "the most basic definition of qualitative research is that it uses *words* as data".

Whilst language and feeling consistently interpenetrate, they are neither identical with nor reducible to each other. Feeling flows into and out of language; it impels talk; it is 'completed' and finessed by (inner) speech; it is (artificially, temporarily) stabilised, communicated and represented in words and phrases. At the same time, language interpellates or 'calls out' feeling, organising experience in accord with regimes of discourse and practice. Sometimes – for example, in the construction of thought and emotion as distinctly separate psychological realms – the effects of these regimes may be so thoroughly embedded that they are difficult to recognise as such. Nevertheless, feeling and language differ in their characteristics and temporalities: the ways that they are able to generate, sustain and communicate meaning are therefore different. Consequently, a wholly linguistic epistemology will not suffice for research into feelings: first, because the meanings, interests and concerns they bear are not representational; second, because the movements, textures, intensities and valences of feeling are known corporeally *before* they are (optionally, imperfectly, temporarily) seized upon linguistically.

An alternative epistemology that places as much weight upon feeling as upon language is provided by Ruthrof (1997), who begins with accounts of meaning that locate its emergence within language (and, indeed, other symbol systems). His account accepts the great significance of language and understands that differences between signs (rather than their intrinsic features) are the basis of their meaning. It also endorses poststructuralist enquiry showing how these differences are bound up with cultural and historical changes. His analysis recognises that the meaning of a sign is always dependent on (other, unarticulated) networks of difference and hence always deferred. Indeed, rather than challenging this position, Ruthrof simply supplements and extends it by proposing that embodied experience can itself be treated as a continuous flux of signs.

Like Langer, and in accord with philosophers such as Merleau-Ponty (2002) and Sheets-Johnstone (1999), Ruthrof recognises that the body's feelings and affordances continuously contribute to how the world appears for us. But rather than treating the body either as object or as subject, or even chiasmically (in Merleau-Ponty's terms) as both, Ruthrof proposes that this embodied aspect of experience can itself be treated as a flow of co-occurring somatic signs. These signs are generated by multiple embodied systems which can be (for example) thermal, gustatory, kinaesthetic or haptic in character. The continuously embodied character of experience means that linguistic signs, with which qualitative research more usually engages, are always already bound up with and suffused by other *embodied signs* in the form of sensations or feelings. In this way, the conventionally meaningful signs of language are never separate from the primordially meaningful signs of the body: what we speak and what we hear is always influenced by how we feel, and vice versa.[3]

However, these felt signs are not fully meaningful in isolation: their meaning always gets interpreted alongside other (typically linguistic) signs. Consequently, their meanings are neither asocial nor simply a matter of social convention. A feeling of anxiety is already meaningful, but we also interpret this feeling – immediately, in the lived moment of its occurrence – to render it thoroughly sensible: we have forgotten something important, we are in a situation that is going to be unpleasant or painful, we are going to be late and so on. Feelings are already endowed with a kind of primordial intentionality derived from their bodily qualities of valence, texture and so on (Geir, 1976). However, their *full* significance must be worked up in conjunction with the meanings of other, co-occurring signs if we are to act upon them appropriately (and even then, of course, our interpretations may be inaccurate).

Equally importantly, Ruthrof is clear that embodied signs are not meaningful *only* because of their interpretation through other sign systems: he rejects the cognitivist claim that feelings and sensations depend solely on context for meaning (a claim often supported with reference to Schacter and Singer's work – see Chapter 3 in this volume). Rather than imagining that embodied signs are entirely meaningless without subsequent interpretation, Ruthrof recognises that they provide intensities, textures, valences and directions that resist some interpretations and promote others: a feeling of pleasure, for example, is not a feeling of anxiety, and nor is it a feeling of pain, sexual desire, thirst, love, nausea, fatigue or satisfaction.

Hence, meaning is never solely linguistic: the signs of language are always already suffused with embodied signs, such that the two always come together. Meaning, therefore, has to be understood as both intersemiotic – constituted by the convergence of two or more sign systems – and heterosemiotic, or heterogeneous, in character. This treatment of feelings as signs provides qualitative researchers with an epistemology that allows them to include language and feeling jointly in their work. In combination with Langer's process ontology of feeling as the raw stuff of experience, Ruthrof's epistemology may facilitate rigorous analyses of qualitative data in ways that reveal its embodied, felt aspects.

## Methodological strategies

Such analyses are also facilitated by the adoption of appropriate methodological strategies, and a range of options have been pursued.

Elsewhere (e.g. Cromby, Brown, Gross, Locke, & Patterson, 2010; Cromby & Phillips, 2014) I have demonstrated how analytics from discourse and conversation analysis can be deployed to examine how interactions are jointly ordered by intertwining patterns of feeling and language. This approach has been called an 'affective-textual analysis', by which is meant not a new method but a re-situating of existing methodological strategies within an alternative conceptual framework. In conversation analysis, Stevanovic and Perakyla (2014) have made a similar move, and (McAvoy, 2015) makes a related argument for her more Foucauldian style of discursive analysis; these strategies can also be related to Wetherell's (2015) call for studies of affective-discursive practices. Another prominent methodological strategy is memory work (Haug, 1987; Crawford, Kippax, Onyx, Gault, & Benton, 1992), which has already been used successfully to explore both emotion and embodiment (Gillies et al., 2004).

At the same time, data derived from sources other than language alone can also generate rich, comprehensive analyses of feeling: analyses of photographs, drawing, paintings, objects, places and walks. Photographs and drawings have been used to investigate embodied experience generally (Gillies et al., 2005) and might be especially appropriate since "the way in which we *live* feelings and experiences are not always available to verbal description" (Reavey & Johnson, 2008, p. 299). Images are sometimes described as facilitating the 'feeling again' of experiences (Radley & Taylor, 2003) and have some potential to evoke – for both researchers and participants – felt understandings that are difficult to convey by using words alone.

Finally, there is still a relatively limited place for quantitative method. Ratner's (2000) argument that quantification is necessary to elucidate the connections between feeling states and social structures suggests that mixed-methods research combining quantitative and qualitative techniques might also sometimes be valuable. Experience sampling of emotionality and mood could be used either to identify participants most suitable for detailed, qualitative investigation, or to add context to case studies or research projects with small samples, and intrinsically 'hybrid' methods such as Q-sorts can also be used to investigate feelings and emotions (Stenner & Stainton-Rogers, 2004).

## Conclusion

Chapter 1 briefly described how, in scholarship associated with the affective turn, affect is frequently positioned as outside and before social meaning, and how critics see this as problematic. For example, Wetherell (2015) argues that it makes little sense either to posit embodied affects arising before and separately from language, or to assume that participants' linguistic accounts of emotion – understood simply *as* accounts – are the only things we can analyse. Nevertheless, whilst Wetherell's position that psychologists should conceptualise and study both feeling and language broadly accords with the arguments developed here, there are sometimes problems with the way such positions are being taken up. First, some researchers are using such arguments to warrant effectively treating emotions as simply 'natural'. Rather than explicitly aligning themselves with sophisticated conceptualisations of emotion such as Burkitt's (2014; see Chapter 3 in this volume) which recognise their historical, cultural and relational contingency, in not theorising them at all some scholars effectively treat emotions as naively humanistic phenomena.[4] Second, emotions and feelings are sometimes analysed only as occasional or episodic intrusions, as though all talk were not already feeling-laden and feeling were not continuous. This style of analysis replicates, albeit implicitly, the illusory cognition–affect divide and plays into the kind of 'depth and surface' dichotomy that Parker (2015) identifies.

Whilst feeling can be approached through language, there is a distance. This means that researchers will always need to be working with an appropriate concept of feeling and cannot simply proceed as though the linguistic alone were adequate to capture its relational patterns, ineffable dynamics and embodied meanings. It implies that, alongside analyses of language, analyses of corporeal practices are also needed, because these practices embed regimes of social influence as enduring patterns, habits or organisations of feeling, in ways that may bypass or contradict overt discursive meanings. The body primordially constitutes experience with feelings that are already socialised, feelings whose socialisation reflects histories of engagement with practices that are only partially linguistic: our methods need to work with this actuality, not to obscure it.

# 6
# Believing

This chapter marks the beginning of a change of emphasis. Whereas the preceding chapters were concerned with feeling in general, this and the next two chapters will show how a focus upon feeling might change how we approach a small set of topics in health and clinical psychology. Although health and illness inescapably involve the body and our experience of it, health psychology resembles psychology generally in being dominated by cognitive studies within which bodies and embodiment are largely discounted. These studies sit alongside biological psychological research where the physicality of the body–brain system and its processes predominate, and psychology is largely reduced to relatively crude inference from the workings of these neural, anatomical and physiological systems. Similar tendencies are also apparent in clinical psychology, where illness is conceived as mental rather than physical but studies also tend to be either cognitive or, alternately, neural/biological – and in either case rarely concerned with the embodied feelings that occupy the liminal space between.

In this context, the concept of belief is an appropriate topic; first, because it is widely used within empirical research where it often appears as a variable or explanatory concept. Second, in health and clinical psychology belief is quite frequently explicitly studied: in the following section, belief will be considered in relation to the purported health benefits of religiosity and spirituality, and with respect to social cognition models such as the theory of planned behaviour. And third, as this chapter will argue, despite frequently being co-opted by the cognitive paradigm, belief is already charged with feeling.

## Belief and health

Belief figures prominently in relation to health and health psychology, both as substantive topic and as theoretical construct. Taking perhaps the most obvious example, as substantive topic belief is integral to both religiosity, "a multi-dimensional variable, which refers to the personal beliefs and experience connected to religion, and includes overt behaviours, beliefs, values and goals, and subjective experiences" (Karademas, 2010, p. 240), and spirituality, a more amorphous concept not necessarily associated with organised religion but typically including "belief in a higher being, the search for meaning, and a sense of purpose or connectedness" (Aukst-Margetic & Margetic, 2005, p. 366).

Evidence for possible connections between health and religiosity/spirituality (R/S) has been accumulating for some time. A review of 91 studies by Chida, Steptoe and Powell (2009) concluded that R/S was associated with reduced mortality in healthy (but not diseased) populations, and that this effect was partially independent of both behavioural factors (e.g. smoking, drinking alcohol) and structural variables such as SES. McCullough, Hoyt, Larson, Koenig and Thoresen (2000) reviewed 42 studies and found that religious involvement was significantly associated with reduced mortality, particularly where measures of public involvement (e.g. church attendance) were used. The reviews by Aukst-Margetic and Margetic (2005) and Chida et al. (2009) both suggest that R/S beliefs are associated with reduced cardiovascular disease. Lower rates of cancer, better overall health and increased life expectancy are also found amongst some religious groups (Koenig, McCullough, & Larson, 2000), outcomes linked primarily to strict dietary and health regimes. With respect to mental health, Aukst-Margetic and Margetic (2005) distinguish between intrinsic religiosity (i.e. for its own sake) and extrinsic religiosity (for pragmatic or instrumental reasons); they find that intrinsic religiosity is associated with a reduced likelihood of being given a diagnosis of depression and with lower levels of anxiety. There is also evidence that physiological processes are modulated by belief: Lissoni et al. (2001) review literature suggesting that 'psycho-spiritual status' enhances immune efficacy, and Koenig et al. (1997) found that religious attendance reduced pro-inflammatory cytokines[1] by small but significant amounts.

Nevertheless, some studies find little or no evidence for positive associations between R/S and health (e.g. Meisenhelder & Chandler, 2002). Where correlations do emerge, Sloan, Bagiella and Powell (1999) highlight poorly designed research, failures to control for multiple comparisons, confounds (e.g. healthier people are more likely to attend religious services) and ethical concerns. Rew and Wong (2006) note a preponderance of cross-sectional research and frequent use of unvalidated, single-item measures or indexical indicators. Reviewing 266 medical articles citing religion, Sloan and Bagiella (2002) concluded that only 17% were relevant to positive health outcomes, and that most studies were methodologically flawed. The relationships between R/S and health might be mediated along various biological pathways by diet, smoking, alcohol consumption, sexual behaviour, better sleep, sympathetic nervous system activity or reduced cortisol (Rew & Wong, 2006; Chida et al., 2009), but there is no consensus regarding which are most influential, and Seeman, Dubin and Seeman's (2003) review concludes that the strongest evidence is for positive effects of meditation upon immune and cardiovascular function. In short, despite some evidence for a small positive association between R/S belief and health, many questions remain.

Taking another obvious example, as a theoretical construct belief is fundamental to the widely used social cognition models of health education and health behaviour: notably the health belief model (HBM: see Rosenstock, 1974), the theory of planned behaviour (TPB: see Azjen, 1985) and the theory of reasoned action (TRA: see Azjen & Fishbein, 1980). The HBM presumes that people have agency and therefore can make good health choices when supplied with correct information, and that whether or not they adopt good health behaviours depends upon their beliefs (1) that they are susceptible to an illness, (2) that it could have serious consequences, (3) that preventive or ameliorative behaviours are available to them and (4) that the benefits of these behaviours outweigh the costs. Belief also figures prominently within the TPB, because each of its three core constructs – attitude, subjective norm and perceived behaviour control – are "underpinned by belief" (Darker & French, 2009, p. 862): beliefs about the consequences and corollaries of changing sedimented activity patterns, normative beliefs about self and others, and beliefs about self-efficacy and environmental factors. TPB research utilises belief elicitation studies, within which population beliefs relevant to the activity of interest are sampled using open-ended questions. The TRA, which extends the TPB by adding variables associated with perceived behavioural control – that is, individuals' beliefs about whether they will actually be able to modify their behaviour – is likewise thoroughly dependent upon belief.

These models continue to be widely used in health psychology (Hagger & Chatzisarantis, 2009), although their validity and utility have been questioned (e.g. Mielewczyk & Willig, 2007; Marks, 2008). Alongside their shared dependency on the concept of belief, these models also share a conception, drawn from rational choice theory, of people as informed, calculating and unemotionally rational. This economic theory makes a series of interlinked assumptions: that individuals are most fundamentally motivated by self-interest; that their behaviours result from ranking preferences and making informed choices between them; that these preferences are fairly stable; and that they are derived from individual appraisals of information (Balbach et al., 2006). These assumptions combine to produce a mechanistic, information-processing version of decision-making which is at odds with typical experience. It was argued in Chapter 2 that the kind of universal rationality implicated here is mythical, and that in actuality persons enact culturally and historically specific local rationalities. Whilst rational choice theory has been influential in many disciplines, then, it has also been critiqued within them: Green and Shapiro (1994) outline its 'pathologies' with respect to political science, Kiser and Hechter (1998) summarise a series of sociological objections, England (1989) offers a feminist critique, whilst Barnes and Sheppard (1992) critique rational choice theory from the perspective of geography. These various critiques detail both evidence and arguments that challenge each of the assumptions that constitute the notion of persons upon which the theory depends. Consequently, some economists are now moving away from this ideologically loaded notion of people as individual, self-interested rational choosers, and adopting other, more environmentally embedded notions of behaviour and choice – albeit that, for the most part, their uptake is no less ideologically inflected (Jones, Pykett, & Whitehead, 2013).

Whilst belief differs in content between R/S and social cognition models, it is nevertheless similar in conceptualisation and it serves related functions. In both cases, it is understood as durable and implicit; as associated with practices, choices and activities; and as bearing personal significance and import. In both, it is deployed to account for ways of acting and talking that persist across situations, and so functions as a kind of organising principle: we know that this person has religious beliefs not just because they say they do – or even *whether* they say they do – but because they regularly attend ceremonies, engage in rituals and religious festivals, induct their children into their faith and so on. Belief therefore appears as a psychological state that motivates, guides, impels, warrants, justifies, legitimates, and that aligns activity with some kind of principle, statement or claim.

It is striking, nevertheless, that in psychology belief is almost never defined. It is omitted from many psychological dictionaries, and it gets used without further specification in the overwhelming majority of theories and empirical studies. And whilst related terms ('schema', 'disposition', 'predisposition') are sometimes used in place of or alongside belief, these too are rarely elaborated. Indeed, this lack of clarity is itself seldom acknowledged, although Jervis (2006) provides some discussion with respect to political psychology. He links belief to evaluations, attitudes and opinion, and observes that many beliefs, even those of a non-religious character, are nevertheless imbued with powerful elements of commitment, or faith. He notes that although different kinds of belief appear to have different functions (to index 'inner' states, urge others toward action, or specify causal relations) each appears to point toward "the inextricable role of emotion in sensible thought" (Jervis, 2006, p. 642).

Many philosophers have also considered belief, providing extended discussions from within particular philosophical systems (e.g. Stich, 1983). Nevertheless, to the extent that there is a general consensus it seems unsatisfactory. One well-regarded summary of key philosophical concepts defines belief as "a propositional attitude" (Honderich, 1995, p. 82), described more fully as a "mental state, representational in character, taking a proposition (true or false) as its content and involved . . . in the direction and control of voluntary behaviour". A belief, then, is an *attitude* toward a statement, claim or proposition. This seems reasonable until we encounter the definition of attitude in the same volume: "any mental state with propositional content. Attitudes, in this sense, include beliefs, desires, hopes and wishes" (Honderich, 1995, p. 64). This circularity sabotages any apparent consensus, suggesting that further investigation is desirable.

This chapter will therefore argue that belief be reconceptualised as *an organisation of socialised feeling, contingently allied to discursive practices and positions*. This conceptualisation accords with relevant uses of belief: non-trivial claims about causal relations, values, preferences and complex states of affairs, rather than trivial claims about perception (e.g. 'I believe this object is a table'). It is also consonant with the view that belief is associated with emotion (Jervis, 2006) and connected to desires, hopes and wishes (Honderich, 1995).

## Social belief

Like the embodied experience of which it is a prominent aspect, thinking is already both individual and social. In this context, discursive psychology (Edwards & Potter, 1992) provides a useful starting point from which to consider the already-social nature of belief, since it understands cognition as practical, discursive activity occurring *between* people in conversation. Rather than treating talk as the mere expression of thought, discursive psychology treats it as the medium within which much thinking occurs. Variability in what people say is consequently not seen as evidence of (cognitive) error, but as a manifestation of the ways in which thinking, understood primarily as debate and argumentation, actually proceeds. Discourse is not merely a reflection of or pathway to cognition but a resource within which socially shared processes of negotiation and disagreement jointly accomplish thinking.

Discursive psychology therefore provides important elements of a powerful alternative to cognitive psychology. It redresses the individualist bias of cognitivism by foregrounding people, situations and activities. It also challenges the mechanistic bias of cognitivism, where variability and disagreement almost inevitably get cast as error, by showing how versions of events and situations get differentially constructed to support arguments and positions. Simultaneously, it relocates the study of thinking from the sterile laboratory to the rich, complex world of newspaper interviews, courtrooms, police cells and telephone advice lines – reminding us that thinking always occurs *somewhere*, in the furtherance of some activity, the pursuit of some goal, or the maintenance of some order of affairs. In discursive psychology, belief – along with other psychological constructs such as attitude, memory and emotion – gets conceptualised and studied linguistically as something mobilised and functional in talk between people: it is "re-specified in terms of situated practices" (Hepburn & Wiggins, 2005, p. 595). The intricate links discursive psychology reveals between belief and everyday conversation clearly demonstrate how treating belief solely as an individual psychological attribute obscures many of the ways in which it is embedded in "meaning, experience, emotion, order, individuality, thought, action, identity, sociality, rationality, symbolism and power" (Day, 2010, p. 10).

Baerveldt and Voestermans (2005) applaud the way that discursive psychology shows how beliefs get constructed in discourse, where they are tailored to specific contexts and used flexibly to manage dilemmas, construct identities, impute responsibility and so on. They note that discursive psychology also engages with the ways that beliefs are rhetorically structured, such that their form already anticipates possible challenges or refutations. This shows how beliefs "do not exist in a social vacuum or in individual human minds", but are "advanced and responded to in the course of ongoing conversational activity, of claims and counterclaims" (Baerveldt & Voestermans, 2005, p. 454).

At the same time, Baerveldt and Voestermans also argue that discursive psychology is incomplete because it cannot adequately explain how people come to jointly invest or 'have faith' in some constructions of the world rather than others:

> The problem, then, is not how our accounts produce 'versions' of the world that can somehow be treated as real, but how, given the almost unlimited range of discursive versions, we can still believe in a shared world, so that we can act in it, rather than just talk about it.
>
> (Baerveldt & Voestermans, 2005, p. 452)

They suggest that discursive explanations of the variability and situatedness of belief in everyday life come at the cost of obscuring the ways in which beliefs can compel and organise activity, and of how they persist across social and material contexts. Discursive psychology's constructionist focus on the local, situated deployment of belief largely conceals its enduring, normative aspects, the ways in which it reproduces (and is reproduced by) larger cultural systems and social hierarchies. This is at least in part because discursive psychology does not adequately consider the felt or affective dimensions of belief. Other scholars have pointed to (versions of) this problem, noting how discursive analyses problematise our understanding of the way that people valorise some identities rather than others (Wetherell, 1995), and how the embodied desires that produce the dilemmas analysed using discursive psychological notions of stake and accountability are paradoxically excluded from its analyses (Willig, 2001). Likewise, using a detailed analysis of a short conversation, Brown and Stenner (2009, pp. 71–76) show how discursive psychology does not adequately consider the shared perceptible world within which conversation always takes place, nor its extraverbal pragmatic situation, omissions which contribute to its inability to properly address the feeling-laden, evaluative aspects of what is said. Despite the advantages of discursive psychology, then, it shares with cognitive psychology a tendency to treat belief solely "as something that is claimed or stated, rather than lived" (Baerveldt & Voestermans, 2005, p. 453).

We can begin treating belief as something that is lived or experienced by first supplementing discursive psychology with an account, such as that given in Chapter 4, of how discourse inhabits individual thought. Vygotsky's (1962) analyses of the acquisition of inner speech show how the conversations that discursive psychology studies provide templates and resources within which, and with which, individual thinking proceeds. Similarly, Billig's (1987) analysis of argumentation and its close links with thinking proposed that thought itself is argumentative or rhetorical in structure, deriving its content and form from successive prior conversations. Like Vygotsky, Billig suggests that we think largely as we talk: thinking is a discussion with oneself that shares features and positions with spoken arguments in everyday life. What we call belief gets worked up rhetorically in discussions that provide both its core content and its nuances. Consequently, Billig (1987, p. 254) suggests that we do not have entirely rigid belief systems: even the most principled, strongly held belief will to some extent get finessed – both in interaction, and in thought – according to occasion, context and situation.[2]

For both Billig and Vygotsky, then, thinking has a conversational aspect and is shaped and maintained in social relations. Uniting their theoretical perspectives with empirical evidence from discursive psychology enables us to work toward an account of belief "that honors the inherent inseparability of the psychological and the social emphasized by discourse-theoretic approaches while positing a (reconceived) 'mental space' as the site of thought processes on a given moment" (Falmagne, 2012, p. 2). It helps explain how individual belief tends to reproduce cultural norms, the precepts, expectations and values of particular times and places (Day & Coleman, 2010). It further suggests how, within such broad cultural patternings, the beliefs of particular individuals are produced through the mediation of their specific history of social relations – with parents, carers, teachers, significant others – with which these acquired norms get inflected.

Beliefs, in other words, display radical individuality. They are constituted within contingent trajectories of relating, the particularities of which inflect their constitution. Whilst two given people might profess belief in the same God, their belief will be differently constituted in accord with factors that include historical epoch, (sub)cultural setting, religion or sect, all of these refracted by the unique, situated, never-to-be repeated ways in which they each encountered these influences. Yet at the same time, their belief in God appears superficially 'the same' precisely because it is constituted from and within shifting combinations of socio-culturally shared discourses, practices, symbols, icons, rituals, settings and situations.

## Felt belief

Experiencing and thinking are not only social, they are also felt. Sharp distinctions between thinking and feeling cannot be sustained, in large part because – as organisms, not machines – it is our continuous capacity to feel that primordially constitutes our thinking. We have seen how Vygotsky's account of the acquisition of inner speech, in a course from conversation through outer speech, can be extended by adding a further stage where feeling comes to stand for inner speech. As fragments of conversation and their corresponding elements of feeling get rehearsed together they become interchangeable: corporeal analogues of meanings, initially borne of conversation, can then get enacted through the body. In this way belief is acquired, not merely as (fragments of) conversation, but also, simultaneously, as an organisation of feeling.

For example, I can articulate both reasons and evidence to support my belief that current UK economic and social policies will damage the health of many thousands of people (for an accessible summary, see Stuckler & Basu, 2013). However, I can also simply experience feelings of anger and mistrust toward the voices of politicians, feelings that arise even before I attend to what they say. Whilst in this instance discourse and practice have inculcated an organisation of feeling, this potential for transformation is bi-directional. My feeling of unease on first meeting someone can subsequently get completed and interpreted – in inner speech, conversation, or both. This will stabilise and sustain my felt disquiet, making it communicable by enabling me to represent it to myself and others, and perhaps culminate in my formalising it as a belief that this person is not to be trusted.

Whilst these examples illustrate that discursive positions can be transformed into organisations of feeling, and vice versa, they do not identify processes whereby these transformations might occur (Falmagne, 2012). The process is essentially one of reconfiguring what is remembered, where previously experienced combinations of discourse and feeling get transformed over time through recall and mobilisation. Repeated linkages between certain phrases, terms and feelings produce habitual associations between them: these associations constitute a web of latent tendencies to feel this, rather than that, in relation to this (rather than that) object, person, place, situation, event, claim or symbol.

This is only possible once we recognise that, psychologically, meaningful claims are never merely linguistic terms. As we hear, read, think or speak them, they are *already* laden with feelings that co-constitute their particular meaning, in that moment, for us. This applies to solitary reading no less than to conversation. Reading is trivially embodied: it requires a brain to co-ordinate activity and register information, eyes to see, hands to hold the book, fingers to turn the page etc. But it is also profoundly embodied, in the sense that engaging with and understanding the text necessarily mobilises embodied sensations, affects and feelings of knowing. Whether verbal or written, language becomes meaningful when individuals endow it with feelings that co-constitute its momentary significances, implications and value. The difference between dead words in an unread text and living words taken up psychologically is that, in the second case, discourse and feeling are already conjoined.

These feelings may include the relatively visceral responses we would identify using emotion terms; they may include extra-emotional feelings that load positions with shades of wanting or avoidance; and they may include logical feelings of knowing – of disjunction, association and so on. None of these types of feelings are necessarily exclusive of the others, and all will reflect the context of discourse as well as its content. Likewise, all may be qualified in ways that reflect the temporal organisation of their enactment: we might *mistrust* a written argument because the author *moves too fast*, feel *impatient* because writing seems *ponderous*, feel *breathless* as a detective novel *races* toward its conclusion and so on. Thus, any meaningful claim, statement or text is already laden with feeling, precisely because this is how *all* meaning is co-constituted (Ruthrof, 1997). Repeated articulations between feelings and their associated discursive practices and positions, contingently organised and interpellated by social relations, then develop the immanent and habitual organisations of feeling that characterise believing.

To summarise so far: (inner) speech is already feeling-laden. Through repetition and rehearsal, speech can therefore inculcate a corresponding organisation of feeling. Just as the transformation from inner speech to feelings of knowing proceeds through subtraction, to produce metacognitive elements of more efficient and general applicability, so in believing there is a process of subtraction within which all unnecessary language can get stripped away to leave an immanent organisation of feeling. Of course, this does not mean that belief can no longer be verbally articulated: simply that its applicability gets broader as its relation to any *specific* discourse becomes more general. In this way, belief can persist across situations and settings associated with a variety of discursive practices and positions, whilst simultaneously remaining discernible as a form of consistency across them.

At the same time, it is important to avoid any implication that belief can *only* be inculcated as the extraneous surplus or residue left behind once language is removed (Falmagne, 2012): corporeal practices can also contribute. Recall that the transformational potentials between feeling and inner speech are bi-directional: in primordially co-constituting experience, feeling impels discourse just as much as, if not more than, discourse interpellates feeling. Caution is needed here, in view of Langer's (1967) observation that those feelings not seized upon by discursive or other representational forms (such as art or musical notation) simply come and go without our ever noticing or recalling them (see Chapter 2): it is only through linguistic or symbolic 'completion' that feelings acquire their full, representational meaning. Nevertheless, Falmagne is correct to emphasise how belief is *already* inculcated corporeally, as well as discursively. Consider how in Orwell's '1984' the 'two minutes hate' – a scheduled time for workers to collectively enact disinhibited public fury at film of 'the enemy' – contributed, alongside re-writing history and controlling the media, to the inculcation of benevolent beliefs about Big Brother and the Party. More disturbingly, Orwell's fictional account has real world counterparts:

> In the US military during certain historical periods, 'hate training' was rampant. Accordingly, during Vietnam, rage at superiors fostered during training was transformed and channelled into fury at the enemy. The 'logic' of such practices was an attempt to demean and debase troops in a manner that could later be directed towards antagonists in Southeast Asia . . . in order to earn self-respect and to enter the military group, the newly mobilised civilian has to adopt new standards. After he has survived basic training, he enters the 'in-group' and then uses the same practices used against him towards others. It is thus reasonable to assume that trainees learn on their very bodies how those who do not belong should be treated.
>
> (Bar & Ben-Ali, 2005, pp. 146–147)

Thus, the repetitions and rehearsals that inculcate belief need not be exclusively or primarily discursive. Feelings that emphasise distinctions between self and others in general can first be rehearsed, encouraged, strengthened and normatively legitimated, in corporeal practices that initially intensify and organise them in relatively inchoate ways and only later direct them in specific ways. The corporeal constitution of these coarsely arranged organisations of feeling primes and constitutes the person as one for whom certain discourse and symbols can subsequently get readily attached, thus to serve as guides, goals or targets.

## Acquiring belief

Belief does not uniquely combine discourse and feeling: it is a particular form of felt thinking, characterised by durability and personal significance. Since its origins are in the social and material circumstances where belief becomes relevant (and, more specifically, within the enactments, repetitions and rehearsals they contain) we can elucidate belief by examining those circumstances. To illustrate this we can consider religiosity, specifically Anglo-American Christianity. The brief analysis that follows is very general, intended to illustrate typical processes of belief formation rather than make specific, grounded claims. It follows others (e.g. Durkheim, 1995 [1912]; Marshall, 2002) that focus on ritual and practice, and echoes Smith (2007) in emphasising the role of feeling in the workings of Christian belief.

Speaking very broadly, then, Christian belief consists of organisations of feeling and associated discourses and narratives developed through various ritualised and frequently overlapping discursive and corporeal practices, including: contemplation, prayer, confession, penitence, abstinence, meditation, clapping, dancing, drumming, swaying, singing and chanting. In varying degrees, these practices discursively invoke hierarchy, ritual and tradition, and may include reading, clothing, costumes, incense, touch, icons, statues, engravings, films, food, drink, immersion in water and other multi-sensorial components. They may also include more mundane (for Durkheim, profane) practices associated with " 'potluck dinners', bingo nights, sports, youth groups, reading groups and 'gossip with friends' " (Smith, 2007 p. 176). They get enacted in multiple settings (home, classroom, church, church hall), some with dedicated architectures and iconographies; associated with both momentous life events (births, deaths, marriages) and with the regular passage of time (Christmas, Easter); and involve variously sized collectives of differentially significant others.

Whilst these multiple, interlocking practices will recruit many different feelings, the Christian tradition frequently emphasises emotional feelings of happiness, love, pride (Tsai, Miao, & Seppala, 2007) and guilt (Albertsen, O'Connor, & Berry, 2006). Christian practices simultaneously marshal feelings of knowing, such as being accepted by others; having confidence in the future; and having arcane or privileged knowledge about reality. They may also recruit extra-emotional feelings of hunger, thirst, satiation, bodily discomfort, touch and sexual desire, and emotional feelings of loneliness, affection, companionship and trust. All these feelings get stabilised by their repetition within rituals imbued with tradition, authority and power; by their relational interpellation in complex mixtures (Scheff, 2003); by effortful engagement with the discursive and corporeal practices that generated them; by the frequently rhythmic character of those practices; and through the mediation of embodied and social processes including heightened arousal, entrainment, social facilitation and de-individuation (Marshall, 2002).

So Christian practices are mediated and organised by multiple objects and settings and enacted through various discursive and corporeal practices, with which, through repetition and rehearsal, the feelings they interpellate get contingently associated. Moreover, these associations are not worked up at exclusively Christian sites since they can also be functional elsewhere – for example, in everyday moral enactments (Smith, 2007). Consequently, they produce somewhat heterogeneous organisations of feeling that nevertheless imbue discourse and narrative with degrees of personal significance; organisations that valorise some discursive constructions and narrative positions rather than others, albeit in variable ways. They may associate particular organisations of feeling with behavioural injunctions ('don't eat fish on Fridays', 'attend church on Sundays'); with discursive regimes of ethics and value that reproduce wider societal structures of difference and power (adultery is a sin; charity is a virtue); and with more abstract or universal discursive constructions ('god', 'divinity', 'soul').

It must be emphasised that this account in no sense denies the significance of Anglo-American Christian belief, which is not diminished by a better understanding of its ontogenesis. It simply demonstrates that what we call beliefs are not so much singular cognitive entities as complex, variegated habits of felt thinking: far more contingent upon the flows of social practice, and far more rooted in our bodies, than psychology usually allows. This can also be illustrated with respect to another example more directly relevant to health: the acquisition of health beliefs related to smoking.

Nicotine smoking impacts upon physiology and can directly influence feeling states: smokers describe extra-emotional feelings of enjoyment, satisfaction, relaxed alertness or concentration, and (where dependency exists) alleviation of the discomfort associated with abstinence (Vangeli & West, 2012). Tobacco companies and advertisers have long worked to exploit these various feelings. With specific reference to women, Anderson, Glantz and Ling (2005) detail how they have systematically associated them with leisure time, relaxation, indulgence, pampering and escape, and with enjoyable social situations, social acceptability, emotional understanding and acceptance. Advertisers have also tried to deliberately combat feelings of guilt and social exclusion amongst smokers, and to associate smoking with slimness, fashionableness, sex appeal, affluence, independence, adventure and exclusivity. Anderson, et al. (2005) show how these efforts are explicitly designed to associate smoking with positive emotional feelings, enabling smokers to experience themselves as 'deserving' (op. cit., p. 128) whilst distancing themselves from notions of smokers as offensive, unlovable, socially unacceptable or different (op. cit., p. 129); they also describe how advertising slogans such as 'Spoil Yourself', 'For People Who Like to Smoke' and 'It's a Woman Thing' crystallise these associations.

Within the framework proposed here, such slogans can be seen as both condensing and mediating particular sets of associations between discourse, feeling and smoking. In Whitehead's (1927) terms, they can be seen as propositions, in the sense that they are 'lures for feeling'.[3] Nevertheless, the beliefs of individual smokers will not look just like these slogans. Instead, they will reflect how the complexes of feeling and discourse the slogans crystallise have been enacted within radically individual concatenations of experience: where smoking has made the person feel good, punctuated a work regime, helped smooth an emotional crisis, alleviated domestic boredom, accentuated a pleasurable moment, or facilitated a social interaction, through social relations where the smoker has come to feel somewhat confident, independent, accepted, exclusive, affluent, attractive and so on.

Each smoker's beliefs will therefore be unique and individual, whilst simultaneously sharing common elements and still being socially and corporeally produced. Moreover, where these beliefs are positive it is not always accurate to simply cast them as irrational. Graham (1987) found that some (predominantly, white) women with children who were living in economically disadvantaged conditions smoked *despite* having adequate knowledge of its adverse health consequences. For these women, smoking was a way of alleviating the combined strains of poverty and parenting, of seizing back moments for themselves, and of managing the various conflicting demands placed upon them:

I smoke when I'm sitting down, having a cup of coffee. It's part and parcel of resting

I think it gives me a break. Having a cigarette is an excuse to stop for five minutes

Smoking calms me down when I get het up and when I've finished something

Sometimes I put him [child] outside the room, shut the door and put the radio on full blast and I've sat down and had a cigarette, calmed down and fetched him in again

Sit down, make a cup of tea, have a cigarette and if she's being really naughty put her in her bedroom and come downstairs.

(Graham, 1987, pp. 52–54)

Graham's study demonstrates that there are situations in which smoking can be understood as a perfectly rational response to social and material circumstances. It also suggests how the vague, alluring promises of advertising can actually gain some traction within the lives of smokers.

More generally, the recognition that feelings are integral to beliefs about smoking illuminates disparate aspects of the literature. It helps explain why smokers persist in smoking despite frequently having adequate knowledge of its dangers (Oncken et al., 2005). In everyday life smoking is often rewarding and facilitative of social interaction, and the feelings it generates may provide ready (im-mediate) disincentives to disregard health warnings. It suggests reasons why nicotine replacement therapy is effective for some (but not all – Silagy et al., 1994) because it temporally separates the extra-emotional feelings of withdrawal from the many other feelings associated with smoking. Similarly, it may help explain why participants in group interventions to help smokers quit frequently mention the significance of various feelings, including attachment to friends, embarrassment at lapsing, feelings of connection, strength and bravery, and feeling a sense of achievement (Vangeli & West, 2012, pp. 176–177).

## Implications

This account has numerous implications for health psychology. Research into R/S and health has predominantly assessed belief using behavioural indicators (e.g. church attendance) and questionnaires. This account demonstrates that both are restricted because what are superficially 'the same' beliefs and activities actually get constituted differently, and have different meanings, according to the particular history of discursive and corporeal practices, the specific narrative positions and organisations of feeling, that they implicate. Potter and Wetherell (1987) observed that forced-choice questionnaires artificially suppress response variation, eliminating 'it depends' and decontextualising responses onto a grid of pre-defined possibilities. With respect to religiosity questionnaires, this restriction extends beyond an inability to reflect nuance and context. Although different respondents might all 'strongly agree' that 'God helps me to lead a better life' (Francis Scale of Attitudes Towards Christianity: Francis, 1993), the meaning of their agreement might differ in accord with the different organisations of feeling each respondent associates with concepts such as 'God'. Within spirituality rituals are typically less formalised, so variation will tend to be correspondingly greater; conversely, even those discourses and organisations of feeling enacted during regular church attendances will vary – from person to person, occasion to occasion. We should not be surprised, therefore, that research using either behavioural indicators or questionnaire indices of R/S generates somewhat variable findings.

To the extent that reviews (e.g. Chida et al., 2009) suggest a small effect of R/S that cannot be accounted for by differential patterns of diet, alcohol consumption, social support and other variables, this account suggests two explanations. First, the feelings integral to belief may have direct consequences: emotions, for example, are implicated in coronary and cardiovascular diseases (Everson-Rose & Lewis, 2005; Ruiz, Hutchinson, & Terrill, 2008) and can modulate immune function (Kiecolt-Glaser, McGuire, Robles, & Glaser, 2002). Religiosity is associated with acceptance of chronic pain (Gerberhagen, Trojan, Kuhn, Limroth, & Bewermeyer, 2008), and pain is a socialised feeling with an emotional component (Rhudy, Williams, McCabe, Rambo, & Russell, 2006). Park (2007) proposes that the associations between R/S and health might be interrogated from a 'meaning systems' perspective where different aspects of belief map onto specific health practices and pathways: this account extends her suggestion by showing how the meanings enacted in belief already implicate embodied processes. Second, many measures used in this research already implicate feeling. Religiosity is positively associated with health-related quality of life (Gerberhagen et al., 2008), a measure that typically includes 'emotional' and 'subjective' well-being subscales. Evidence suggests that positive affect is associated with good health (although this research suffers from similar problems to research into R/S – Pressman & Cohen, 2005): to the extent that the organisations of feeling interpellated by R/S belief are also hedonically positive, this might be largely the same effect viewed from a different perspective.

This account also has wider implications, with regard to the typical conceptualisation of belief – in the HBM, the TPB, the TRA, and indeed elsewhere in psychology – as a discrete, cognitive variable. Belief is discursive before it is cognitive: its cognitive aspects are secondary to the social, discursive practices that engendered them. Moreover, this social influence does not end once belief is acquired: belief remains continuously social, an element of the 'boundary phenomena' that Shotter (1993) identifies. Far from being rigidly demarcated and cognitive, belief is enacted and influential in ways that continuously reflect the ebb and flow of feeling within the contingency, multiplicity and variability of everyday life.

It has been well established that this variability remains relevant even when it is artificially minimised by psychological research procedures. Surveys and experiments are particular, unusual social situations (Wyer, 1974), and Mielewczyk and Willig (2007) review evidence indicating that this causes problems for two of the TPB's three component variables, subjective norms (SN) and perceived behavioural control (PBC). Even when measures of SN and PBC are supplemented with or replaced by others, to increase their explanatory power, studies using the TPB typically account for only 42–44% of variance in intended outcomes (McEachan, Conner, Taylor, & Lawton, 2011), whilst recent meta-analyses have found that the TPB only predicts between 36% (Trafimow, Sheeran, Conner, & Finlay, 2002) and 19.3% (McEachan et al., 2011) of variance in actual behaviour change. Mielewczyk and Willig (2007) suggest that these disappointing results are in part because the 'health behaviours' targeted by social cognition models do not actually exist as discrete categories of activity. As we saw in Chapter 2, the meaning of, for example, not using a condom is relationship and circumstance dependent, and not simply calculable in terms of 'objective' health risks (Willig, 1995).

Simultaneously, Balbach et al. (2006) show how the notion of persons as self-interested, isolated and rational appraisers of information – upon which these social cognition models depend – has been used by the tobacco industry to deflect responsibility for the disease and illness their products cause. The industry frequently claims that its only societal duty is to provide neutral information to assist consumers in making their own rational choices, and this helps it evade calls for more meaningful forms of corporate social responsibility. This notion of persons as rational choosers can be contrasted with a notion of persons whose felt experience is consistently embedded in dynamic matrices of social relations and material circumstances, persons for whom the appraisal of information about the health dangers of tobacco is never simply separate either from their embodied experiences of smoking it or from the social and material circumstances they occupy.

Whilst similar processes underlie the acquisition of both health and R/S beliefs, there are also marked differences between them because repetition, rehearsal, performance and formalised ritual loom considerably larger in R/S. There are undoubtedly elements of repetition in the acquisition of health beliefs: repeated exposure to advertising, to the views of others, to feelings of pain, fatigue, discomfort, nausea, dizziness, to situations within which a cigarette has felt good, not using a condom has been rewarding and so on. However, these repetitions are less formalised, less homogeneous, and less consistently associated with specific icons and symbols. By contrast to R/S beliefs, this means that health beliefs are likely to be more informal, dispersed and internally contradictory. Santiago-Delefosse (2012) suggested that these differences might ultimately lead us to question whether the term 'belief' is actually appropriate. In working with health beliefs, social science and psychology have drawn folk psychological notions of belief into research without first seriously interrogating them. It may be that habitual associations between discourse, practice and feeling which are not ritualistically inculcated, and which consequently remain less formalised and more disaggregated, are better described using another term such as 'sensibilities' (Cromby, 2012).

This account does illustrate that to treat belief as solely discursive would be to erroneously reduce it to something claimed or stated, rather than something lived. Alongside its discursive-cognitive aspect belief is an organisation of feeling that enacts and reproduces personally held, socially obtained values. Belief therefore tends to reproduce wider social divisions and their associated power relations, and recognising this allows us to investigate its character in relation to socio-economic, cultural and political conditions (Marks, 2008). 'Health beliefs' arise as moments or acts within ongoing social-embodied processes, continuously and contingently mediated by bodies, discourses, practices, resources, objects and places.

## Conclusion

The notion that belief includes an organisation of feeling alongside and within its discursive instantiations challenges the overly rational and individualistic notion of belief circulating within cognitive psychology and related spheres. The status of belief as an amalgam of feeling and discourse suggests, since feelings are a-representational, ineffable and constitutive of experience, that we might not always wholly know what or even *that* we believe.[4] Belief, in its felt aspect, might sometimes hover on the fringes of awareness, sometimes perceptible and sometimes implicit (but nevertheless consistently influential). Moreover, whilst some characteristics of individual belief can be attributed to parental or family dynamics, this chapter has shown how circuits of social and material influence, enacted through discursive and corporeal practices, are equally significant.

Belief arises when social practice works up organisations of feeling in contingent association with discourse and practice. Consequently, beliefs are enduring, yet variable and flexible; they have largely predictable content, yet are contingent upon the actions and talk of others; they are social, yet can be endowed with deep personal significance. Believing is not merely information-processing activity, and belief is not an individual cognitive entity. Belief is the somewhat contingent, socially co-constituted outcome of repeated articulations between discourses, narratives, corporeal practices and feelings. In a second-order process, a work of social construction parasitic upon this co-constitution, belief is also a category of both lay and academic psychological discourse. Psychology has little to lose, and something to gain, by engaging with these processes of co-constitution.

# 7
# Exhausting

This chapter engages with an issue briefly touched upon in relation to beliefs: how we should conceptualise organisations of feeling, discourse and corporeal practice that – in contrast to those associated with spirituality and religion – are not produced through tightly codified or formalised interactions, nor consistently associated with specific sites, iconographies, texts and rituals. It was suggested that instead of belief we might adopt the term *sensibility*. In this chapter, the example of chronic fatigue syndrome (hereafter, CFS) will be used to show how a particular sensibility might be acquired by some people given this diagnosis.

The analysis rests upon a set of overlapping arguments, including Hacking's (2006) claim that medical and psychiatric diagnostic classifications – by organising the experiences and understandings both of people who receive them and of those who encounter or work with those people – can in a sense function to 'make up' those to whom they are applied (for a version of the present analysis more specifically aligned with Hacking's claim, see Cromby, 2015). In a conceptually related argument, Corcoran (2009) emphasises the significance for social psychology of what he calls our 'second nature' – the acquired, embodied, largely implicit or pre-reflective orientation to self, others and world from within which we approach every situation. Amongst other sources, Corcoran draws upon Shotter's work to argue that this orientation exceeds, enables and yet is bound up with discursive representation.

In the following section, a short discussion of CFS describes the status and features of this diagnosis. This is followed by an analysis of Internet information about the condition. The analysis interweaves consideration of patient's corporeal practices in CFS with analysis of the discursive, rhetorical organisation of information about their condition, information given meaning by the bodily signs they experience. It identifies ways in which some (and *only* some) patients might enact specific corporeal practices, associated with the meanings carried in information about CFS, and shows how these combine to produce a particular sensibility.

## Chronic fatigue syndrome

CFS is a contentious diagnosis, such that even the name of the condition is challenged. Alternatives such as myalgic encephalopathy (ME) or chronic fatigue and immune deficiency syndrome (CFIDS) have been championed, and abusive terms such as 'yuppie flu' rejected. The terminology used here reflects the view that CFS is – perhaps – the least problematic term in current use. Whichever term is used, it indexes a variable, fluctuating pattern of symptoms typically including severe fatigue and persistent, widespread pain (National Institute for Clinical Excellence, 2007). CFS is by definition a chronic condition, lasting at least six months and often enduring for many years, or recurring at intervals over decades: hence its cost, to individuals and services, is considerable.[1]

The embodiment of CFS is sustained, multiple and variable, but elusive. It is typified by an absence of medical signs and a wide variety of symptoms that are distressing, disabling, but on a continuum with 'normal' experience. Together with its disputed status, these characteristics foreground socio-cultural resources, interactional processes and struggles over meaning. A study of the stigmatisation associated with CFS (Jason et al., 2001) showed how its meanings vary as a function both of diagnostic terminology and professionals' disciplinary background. Three versions of the same case history, alternately described as CFS, ME or 'Florence Nightingale Disease', were presented to undergraduates and medical students. Medical students were significantly more likely both to view the illness as serious and consider it a form of psychiatric illness; participants presented with the 'ME' version were significantly more likely to attribute biomedical causation.

CFS is sometimes described as a somatising condition associated with psychiatric diagnoses of depression and anxiety disorder. Within psychiatry, the diagnostic criteria for depression already index significant elements of anxiety (American Psychiatric Association, 2013). It is widely accepted amongst specialists in this field that people given a diagnosis of generalised anxiety disorder cannot be differentiated reliably from those given a diagnosis of depression (Stein & Rauch, 2008), and co-morbidity between these diagnoses is so extensive that some (e.g. Tyrer, 2001) have argued for a mixed 'cothymic' diagnosis. Largely independently of these debates, CFS is sometimes characterised as a form of 'paradoxical' or 'anxious' depression (Sharpe et al., 1997; Hyland, 2002), a view which inhabits both lay and professional reasoning (Horton-Salway, 2004; Guise, Widdicombe, & McKinlay, 2007). Nevertheless, both in academic writing (Wendell, 1996) and everyday talk (Horton-Salway, 2001, 2004; Tucker, 2004; Guise, et al., 2007) CFS patients largely favour its construction as a physical illness and reject notions of psychiatric disorder.

This might suggest that the ME label is preferable, because it is more readily seen to imply biomedical than psychological causation. However, some patients reject this, too, because it creates potentials for CFS to be known as the *me* disease and "might invite more ridicule from critics who tend to portray patients with CFS as self-centred complainers" (Jason et al., 2001, p. 69). Studies of personality in relation to CFS present a stereotype of patients as "perfectionist, conscientious, hardworking, somewhat neurotic and introverted . . . with high personal standards, a great desire to be socially accepted and . . . a history of continuously pushing themselves past their limits" (Geelen et al., 2007, p. 885). However, although they acknowledge that chronic illness can engender personality changes, Geelen et al. (2007) find considerable heterogeneity between CFS patients and no consistent evidence for a widespread constellation of unique personality characteristics. They attribute this in part to the prevalence of cross-sectional designs, and to considerable variability in measures, populations, control groups and case definitions. Whilst they advocate a greater focus upon the illness narratives of patients given a CFS diagnosis, the persistence of this stereotype, and its frequent association with difficult consultations and 'heartsink' patients (Werner & Malterud, 2003), thus remains unexplained.

The empirical data analysed were sampled from the Internet. Studies increasingly show that medical patients use the Internet to find out about their illnesses (Eaton, 2002), including both life-threatening illnesses such as cancer (Ziebland et al., 2004) and conditions like CFS (Asbring & Narvanen, 2004). As the online world has become increasingly entangled with the physical world, Internet content has become less clearly distinguishable from content derived from other sources. Indeed, rather than being distinctively 'new', Internet health information is frequently aligned with that of 'old' media, not least because many content providers strive for cross-platform consistency (Seale, 2005). Nevertheless, what the Internet yields might not be representative so much as indicative, constituting a body of information that is influential simply because, for many, it is readily accessible.

## Method

A Google search for "CFS ME UK" was conducted, and relevant material from the first three pages of hits was downloaded: 18 different websites were included.[2] In order to identify a putative sensibility associated with CFS, a thematic analysis (Braun & Clarke, 2006) was first conducted. Duff (2003, p. 176) observes that "the social and psychological effects of living with CFS derive from ... the physical symptoms of the disease, the cultural response to fatiguing illnesses, and the efforts the sick make to stretch lives worth living between these circumstances". The content of the websites was taken as providing an adequate enough description of the physical symptoms of CFS. The possible efforts made by the sick as a consequence of these symptoms were then identified with respect to the themes identified in the analysis. These themes orient people towards common underlying meanings, encourage them to engage in certain corporeal practices, and so incite them to enact similar kinds of relationships to themselves and others. The identification of what can be seen as 'reasonable' ways of responding to these meanings therefore indicates one kind of sensibility – one way to 'stretch lives worth living' – associated with CFS.

Importantly, this sensibility is neither ubiquitous amongst people with a CFS diagnosis, nor exclusive to them. On the one hand this is because information about CFS is heterogeneous, and because people will inevitably act upon it in somewhat disparate ways. On the other hand, this is because the felt experiences the information is used to interpret are highly variable, so the salience of particular details will both differ and change. Consequently, there will inevitably be variation in the sensibilities associated with CFS, alongside overlap with sensibilities possibly associated with other chronic conditions. The analysis identifies a set of recurring textual meanings and feelings, and a set of corporeal practices reasonably associated with them: jointly, these constitute a sensibility. But this sensibility is therefore *modal*, in the statistical sense of representing the highest peak in what might be a wide and irregular distribution. Rather than identifying an average or mean sensibility in CFS (if this were even meaningful), the analysis merely represents a particular sensibility likely to manifest relatively frequently.

## Analysis

The websites primarily favour the influence of physical factors in the onset and maintenance of CFS. Whilst keenly aware of the conflictual status and chequered history of the condition, they nevertheless imply that CFS is a 'real' (i.e. organic) disease. Consonant with this orientation, they portray CFS as something arising within individuals, for which they must take responsibility by re-ordering their lives to manage and reduce symptoms. However, this internal, physical construction co-exists with another of CFS as exacerbated or 'triggered' by undue activity (too much, or of the wrong kind), or by 'stress', life events, and other illnesses. Simultaneously, the websites bear witness to the uncertainty surrounding the condition. Uncertainty was often most pronounced with respect to causality, although variation in symptoms, course, duration and prognosis, and the variable, inconsistent effects of treatments, were much remarked upon. These uncertainties were typically checked by boundaries drawn between CFS and 'ordinary' tiredness, depression and other diagnoses. CFS was thus constructed as a unique, albeit indistinct, constellation of symptoms, associated with an unspecified physical pathology. These observations, and the practices they legitimate, will be described in more detail in relation to three themes: uncertain physicality, responsibility and balance, and boundaries and conflict.

## Uncertain physicality

Although CFS is constructed as distinctively physical, this physicality is uncertain in relation to causes, symptoms and (although this aspect will not be detailed here) prognoses. Consequently, claims of physicality are typically implied, rather than explicitly stated, and are in constant tension with other readings that threaten to sabotage or contradict them.

### Causes

'Origin' stories are powerful rhetorical devices that situate phenomena intertextually with respect to established conceptual frameworks

(Haraway, 1996). Establishing causality in CFS would generate an effective origin story, strongly supporting its status as organic condition. This may be why, although all the websites acknowledge that causality is unknown, they frequently deploy discursive strategies that imply physical causation without ever stating it:

> For many people, CFS begins after a cold, bronchitis, hepatitis, or an intestinal problem.. For some, it follows a bout of infectious mononucleosis.
>
> (Psychnet, para 13)
>
> Some people will appear to get CFS following a viral infection, or a head injury, or surgery, excessive use of antibiotics, or some other traumatic event.
>
> (CFS news, para 117)

In these extracts, as elsewhere, temporal contiguity suggests a link between other definitively physical conditions and CFS, implying a causal sequence without actually specifying any mechanism or pathway, and claims are further hedged (Hyland, 1996) by referring them only to 'many', or even 'some'. In the second excerpt the phrase 'will appear to get' helps construct CFS as corollary to infectious disease, but avoids definitiveness by referring solely to appearances, suggesting an organic cause whilst avoiding a potentially disprovable claim.

Simultaneously, these implications of physical causality are sabotaged by the great diversity of possible causes, since their sheer number and variety undermine the idea of CFS as singular, unitary and coherent. The extracts above begin to illustrate this multiplicity, which also includes: immune system dysfunction, disruption of biorhythms, irregularities of the hypothalamic-pituitary-adrenal axis, failure of steroid production by the adrenal glands, abnormalities in pituitary gland function, viral causes, deficiencies of B12 or NADH (nicotinamide adenine dinucleotide) and 'genetic factors'.

So far, physical causality is uncertain in two senses: first, it is implied rather than asserted, suggested rather than proven; second, it is multiple and diverse, distributed across a dizzying range of influences. However, it is also uncertain in the sense that the rhetorical work needed to achieve such implications is often accompanied by blunt acknowledgements that causality is actually unknown – even though, as in the extract below, such statements often appear adjacent to others that serve to dilute their impact:

> The cause or causes of M.E. are not fully understood. It often develops after a virus, like flu or glandular fever.
>
> (AFME, paras 20–21)

Such explicit acknowledgements that physical causality is unknown typically legitimate discussion of other influences that, through the mediating effects of stress, lead to illness:

> certain key events – stress, infections, more life events – may precipitate the onset of the illness
>
> (Kings College, para 36)

> High-stress events sometimes seem to 'trigger' the first appearance of the illness and they will usually worsen the symptoms if the illness has already developed
>
> (Netdoctor, para 248)

In biomedicine, stress indexes a diverse range of social, psychological, emotional and biological processes (Brown, 1996) and it has long been established that the common-sense relationship between stressful life events and illness is by no means straightforward (Dohrenwend & Dohrenwend, 1974). Some see stress as an intrinsically reductionist explanatory device (Newton, 2007), and in lay discourse it gets alternately invoked as cause, process and outcome in ways not necessarily consistent with biomedical understandings (Mulhall, 1996). So the uncertainty surrounding CFS is managed, in part, by invoking another construct whose status and boundaries are also unclear.

The invocation of stress also broadens and diffuses causality from the merely physical into the wider realm of experience which is, inevitably, bound up with the vagaries of everyday life. As in the excerpts above, metaphors such as 'triggering' (evoking a sudden, damaging discharge), or 'precipitation' (releasing something already latent) are frequently deployed to manage the further uncertainty raised by suggesting causal associations between mind and body. Both metaphors construct CFS as an already existing entity, awaiting activation – although, paradoxically, both do so by extending causality into the psychological realm. So a further sense in which physical causality is uncertain is that it isn't just physical: the inclusion of life events, emotion and stress extends causality into the realm of relationships, emotions, thoughts and feelings.

## Symptoms

Symptoms are uncertain, firstly, in that they are universally acknowledged to include a striking variety of experiences:

> extreme exhaustion, muscle pain and a severe flu-like malaise... difficulties with concentration and memory, loss of balance, digestive problems, visual disturbances, sleep disorders and mood swings
> (Support ME, para 7)

As this excerpt illustrates, CFS symptoms have three notable characteristics: they often consist primarily of feelings and therefore are mostly invisible, apparent only if commented on or made relevant; they are largely on a continuum with 'everyday' feelings and experiences, making the boundary between symptom and non-symptom a matter of degree, not kind; and they are non-specific, potentially associated with or caused by many other illnesses (and, in their everyday form, no illness at all). They are also acknowledged to be highly variable:

> It is quite possible to have CFS and not have all of these symptoms – an individual's experience of CFS is essentially unique.
> (Netdoctor, para 35)

Variability exists both between and within patients, such that each sufferer's experience is 'essentially' unique – a rhetorical formulation which superficially accentuates uniqueness, but actually moderates it. Uncertain physicality with regard to symptoms resides in their variety, their invisibility, their location on continua with everyday experience, and their variable, gradual or cyclical character.

Symptoms are where the body itself 'speaks', co-constituting the meaning of illness with its own unsought contribution, and the variety and variability of CFS symptoms powerfully instructs patients in the uncertainty of CFS through the medium of their own feeling bodies. By default, bodies go largely unnoticed; they are the necessary but ineffable background of activity, the "darkness needed in the theatre to show up the performance" (Merleau-Ponty, 2002, p. 115). In CFS, however, there is the continuous potential for the body to 'dys-appear' – to appear in a dysfunctional manner (Leder, 1990) – because almost any less-than-pleasant feeling is, potentially, the onset of another symptom.

So CFS gets constructed as an illness caused by elusive and possibly multiple physical influences, the phenomenology of which is highly variable and consists primarily of a range of adverse feelings. What corporeal practices might patients reasonably adopt to manage this uncertainty? One response would be vigilant monitoring of each successive felt bodily state. This suggestion in no way implies uniformity: patients could monitor their feelings conscientiously, intermittently, enthusiastically, guardedly, surreptitiously or ironically, and their monitoring may be infused with feelings of hope, resignation, determination grim desperation and so on. Nevertheless, the requirement to manage a diversity of uncertain causes seems likely to lead some people given this diagnosis to conduct continuous, mindful surveillance of their own feelings: a corporeal practice that can be called somatic monitoring.

Because of its distinctive phenomenological characteristics somatic monitoring seems especially likely when symptoms include extra-emotional feelings of pain. Pain demands attention, constricts spatial awareness to the body and temporal awareness to the immediate moment, and makes its relief the primary focus of intentions (Leder, 1990). However, many other feelings are also implicated: Fennell (2003) associates CFS with trauma and observes that alongside extra-emotional feelings of tiredness and pain it frequently includes emotional feelings of fear, anxiety, grief, anger, sadness and guilt. She observes that diagnosis and illness-acceptance amongst patients are also accompanied by a range of feelings including fear, sadness and loss.

Whilst practices of somatic monitoring might help manage combinations of adverse feelings, they also interpellate feelings of their own. Whereas repeated failures to manage or avoid symptoms may be associated with feelings of distress, feelings of self-efficacy and acceptance in CFS are associated with increased wellbeing (Van Damme Crombez et al., 2006). Similarly, Findley et al. (1998) found that feelings of mastery or self-efficacy amongst CFS patients were related to effective symptom management and lower disability and distress.

So the continuous potential of the body to dys-appear could encourage, for some patients, a corporeal practice of closely monitoring their feelings. At the same time, we have seen how patients are advised that symptoms can be 'triggered', not just by their bodies, but by external events, activities and relationships and the stress these may cause. This could reasonably lead some patients to extend the practice of somatic monitoring in order to regulate these activities and events. Alongside somatic monitoring and its intense focus on bodily states, this suggests a further corporeal practice that can be called experiential regulation: the deliberate ordering of relationships, work and family, and the arrangement and conduct of the minutiae of everyday life, to limit exposure to activities and events that may cause or exacerbate symptoms.

There is evidence suggesting that some CFS patients do enact such practices. Houdenhove and Luyten (2008) listed somatic hypervigilance/pre-occupation as a perpetuating factor in CFS, whilst Knoop et al. (2010) found that tendencies to attend to fatigue and related symptoms, pessimistic beliefs about fatigue and activity, and hypervigilance for fatigue-related cues were all implicated in CFS. Both somatic monitoring and experiential regulation could contribute to the appearance of neurosis amongst patients, and Geelen et al.'s (2007) strongest evidence for a consistent personality trait in CFS was for increased levels of neuroticism. Indeed, the stereotype of CFS patients sketched by Geelen et al. (2007) also includes perfectionism, conscientiousness, introversion and high standards: all characteristics which might be inferred, interpersonally, as the consequence of enacting these two practices.

## Responsibility and balance

Two-thirds of the websites offered advice concerning the management of CFS, from which inter-related themes of responsibility and balance were drawn. Responsibility indexes the manifold ways in which patients should be accountable for the ordering and amount of everything that might impinge upon their condition; balance is the organising principle by which responsibility should be enacted.

## Responsibility

As the diversity of causes and symptoms suggests, the activities, substances and experiences for which patients should be responsible are multiple, variable and heterogeneous. But despite the enormity and imprecision this implies, CFS patients are clearly told that responsibility is theirs:

> You can make a huge difference to how quickly you get better
>
> (Dr Ruth, para 53)

> Self help is vital
>
> (BBC Ask Doctor, para 15)

As these extracts suggest, responsibility is constituted almost exclusively as individual responsibility. The double emphasis on 'you' in the first excerpt accords with the use of 'self' in the second: in both, the self that is implicated is a lone, transcendent one engaging in disciplinary practices of 'self help' that work to align desires and wishes with normative prescriptions regarding subjectivity and the social order (Rimke, 2000).

With regard to the practices by which responsibility should be enacted, most frequently people are simply told to avoid experiences and situations that might induce or exacerbate symptoms. However, suggestions also go beyond the merely negative:

> You should have a careful timetable you must stick to, resting regularly even if you are not tired. This will help to stop you getting a 'relapse' after you exercise. You must not be surprised if you have phases of feeling tired and achy when you start to build up what you do – and you must not let it put you off your timetable.
>
> (Dr Ruth, para 50)

> Hold on to hope, but be prepared for the illness to last a long time
>
> (AFME All About ME, para 168)

Not only must time, exercise and rest be carefully managed, patients must also manage feelings and thoughts: maintaining optimism, avoiding surprise, anticipating tiredness and pain, stoically maintaining discipline and hope. Responsibility includes regimes of feeling and thinking, as well as activity and behaviour, and – as Hacking's (2006) analyses suggest – even imply wholesale reconstruction of the person:

> You will need to take the time to create a new self image for yourself, to know that your new physical limitations do not limit you as a person, as a soul, no matter what other people are thinking.
>
> (CFS News, para 327)

This advice separates 'self' from physicality in ways that contradict other aspects of the information, whilst simultaneously re-emphasising the individual. In a version of the 'magical voluntarism' described by Smail (2005), it is as though becoming who we are is a function of some mysterious inner force of willpower that can be called upon entirely separately from relationships, personal biographies, resources and material circumstances. CFS patients are advised to view their condition as able to strike from any direction, at any moment; to see it as enduring for extended periods, and impacting significantly upon lifestyle: and then advised to take sovereign responsibility for managing this state of affairs.

In positioning patients as vitally culpable agents within the trajectory of their illness, such advice could further entrench corporeal practices of somatic monitoring and experiential regulation. It also engenders paradoxes and dilemmas, since many changes are simply beyond the reach of most patients. For the great majority, responsibility for the temporal quality and affective texture of everyday life cannot be theirs alone: other people, and institutions such as welfare agencies, the medical profession and employers, will always be influential. The degree of responsibility most patients might take is limited by the exigencies of materiality and social structure, but these limitations are elided and an individualised version of the patient as sovereign agent gets constructed. The advice is infused with neoliberal precepts that use notions of 'health promotion' and 'choice' to devolve responsibility for wellbeing to individuals, sidestepping the contribution of social deprivation (Galvin, 2002) and conferring responsibility for health upon individuals (Read, 2009).

## Balance

When patients are told how to *be* responsible, the notion of balance is frequently central. Balance refers to all the ways in which everyday life might impinge upon and exacerbate illness:

> [patients] will often talk in terms of a tightly rationed energy budget. They have so much energy to divide between, say, shopping, keeping on top of the housework and looking after their family. Any increase in expenditure in one area takes precious reserves from another. Unexpected demands – life events, applying for benefits, other illness, relationship problems – can wipe out existing reserves at a stroke. Only by very carefully pacing themselves can they maintain their current commitments.
>
> (Kings College, para 63)

So balance, too, extends into all areas of life. Exhortations of balance also refer more specifically to attempts to alleviate CFS symptoms, particularly with respect to the continuum between resting and exercise where too much of either is presented as troublesome. So balance is not merely about absorbing information – it must be instilled through the deliberate rehearsal of corporeal practices:

> The key to recovery is usually learning to be consistent about what you do – both resting and doing things. Before you can make any

real progress, you will need to learn not to 'yo-yo' between taking too much rest when you are tired or overdoing exercise when you do have energy.

(Dr Ruth, para 45)

Balance might well be an effective organising concept for therapeutic interventions. Barlow, Wright, Turner and Bancroft (2005) found increased self-efficacy and reduced distress at 12-month follow-up after a trial of self-management techniques in CFS, and – as Goudsmit et al. (2012) observe – practices of this kind (e.g. 'pacing') are acceptable to patients. Nevertheless, the forms of self-management they implicate closely resemble the corporeal practices of somatic monitoring and experiential regulation described above, suggesting that these could get further ingrained by attempts to achieve balance.

### Boundaries and conflict

Given that the uncertainty surrounding CFS is acknowledged the websites must orient towards it, and this means asserting boundaries: then, because these boundaries are often contested, issues of conflict also arise.

### Boundaries

CFS patients are constructed as a unity by asserting various boundaries – for example between CFS and fibromyalgia, multiple chemical sensitivity, Gulf War syndrome and Lyme disease. However, the boundary most frequently constructed is between CFS and 'ordinary' fatigue:

The severity and impact of the symptoms experienced by the majority of people with CFS is vastly greater than the symptoms of what one might call 'ordinary' fatigue.

(Netdoctor, para 12)

it is common for between one-third to half the population to experience fatigue when they are run down, but this is very different to the debilitating fatigue experienced by ME/CFS sufferers.

(Support ME, para 8)

In the first excerpt, a rhetorically weak global assertion of difference is avoided by invoking quasi-medical dimensions of 'severity' and 'impact'. In the second, an authoritative statement about the incidence of 'ordinary' fatigue supports the claim that fatigue in CFS is worse. In both, fatigue in CFS is rhetorically demarcated from ordinary fatigue, so constructing a version of this everyday feeling as a symptom.

Another boundary frequently marked is between CFS and depression. The boundaries of depression are themselves fluid and contestable (Thomas-Maclean & Stoppard, 2004) but, like other psychiatric diagnoses, depression is particularly stigmatising (Sayce, 1998). Consequently, the rhetoric employed here is of a different order:

> Many emerging illnesses, before they have gained acceptance by the medical community, have initially been discounted as being hysteria, depression, somatoform disorders, etc. One hundred years ago, polio was dismissed in just that fashion...the finding by Demitrack that cortisol levels are low in CFS patients whereas in depressed people they are high, indicates that CFS is not depression...CFS patients tend to overestimate their abilities, retain a strong interest in life, and respond poorly to exercise, whereas the opposite are typically observed in people who are depressed.
>
> (CFS News, paras 275–276)

The distinction between depression and CFS rests upon various facts (from history, physiology and behaviour) and their detailed deployment does important rhetorical work (Potter, 1996). The authority of an implied academic citation adds weight, as does the way current knowledge is positioned as superior, whilst simultaneously implying physical causality through the comparison with polio. As in previous extracts, physical causality is again suggested rather than claimed, and the arguments are inflected with a lay version of what Woolgar and Pawluch (1985) call 'ontological gerrymandering': the tendency to selectively apply scepticism to some phenomena rather than others.

Demarcating 'everyday' fatigue from the debilitating fatigue of CFS re-affirms its physicality by highlighting a symptom central to its nature. Similarly, distinguishing depression from CFS wards off the stigma of mental illness and, via the cultural commonplace of mind–body dualism, implies physical causation (if it is not one, it must be the other). Nevertheless, because the construction of both boundaries depends upon self-report, CFS patients face the repeated dilemma of persuading others that their feelings of tiredness are different and worse, whilst also – if they are to be entirely believable – effacing any apparent stake in the outcome. Similarly, in circumstances where anyone might feel miserable they must ward off suggestions that they are simply miserable, asserting instead that their problems are organic and their feelings of misery epiphenomenal, not causal.

The frequent reappearance of these dilemmas across multiple sites and social relations presents patients with responsibility for the presentation, as well as the management, of their condition. For some, this might add a further, self-conscious twist to the corporeal practice of experiential regulation, such that they also attempt to influence how they are perceived by others – to regulate other people's experience of *them*, as well as regulating their own activities.

### Conflict

In the construction of disease the assertion of boundaries is associated with conflict (Segal, 1988), and in CFS the absence of diagnostic signs has contributed to medical scepticism regarding its status (Banks & Prior, 2001). Nevertheless, most websites stated that the status of CFS is now accepted: positioning them as modern and well-informed, and those who disagree as ignorant or behind the times. Sometimes, however, continuing disagreement – and variation in medical provision – was explicitly acknowledged:

> Uncertainty about the cause of the condition and effective treatment leads to frustration amongst adult and child patients who may suffer debilitating ill health over a number of years. Patient groups are dismayed by misunderstandings and prejudice which they believe surround the illness and have engendered a climate of disbelief which adds to the distress experienced by the sufferer.
>
> (House of Commons rp98–107, para 27)

The great power of medicine makes conflict over the status of CFS relevant for patients and helps explain why the websites frequently engage in various forms of rhetorical work. Alongside efforts to construct boundaries around CFS, rhetoric is deployed to imply physical causality, to manage the range of competing explanations, and to make what might otherwise be seen as everyday experiences count as symptoms. By definition, rhetoric involves the prior formulation of an argument or claim in such a way as to ward off potential criticism or defend against an alternative position. So these rhetorical strategies, by constructing CFS in a particular way, could function simultaneously to sensitise people to the uncertain, conflicted status of their condition, because the posture they model – the way of talking, arguing about, reflecting upon and accounting for CFS that they present – is one with conflict at its core.

Some patients might therefore be drawn towards a corporeal practice that can be called pre-emptive defensiveness: the feeling-laden performance of a defensive relational stance whereby they protect or assert the reality of their illness before it is ever questioned. This practice could extend not only to demarcating the boundaries of their condition, but to the way people with CFS unthinkingly or habitually talk about their problems in general. Like the other practices described here, pre-emptive defensiveness should not be conceptualised homogenously: it could variously be imbued with emotional feelings of anger, sadness, hostility or impatience, and with feelings of knowing ranging from calm assurance and acceptance, through incomprehension or curiosity, through to feelings of alienation, marginalisation or despair.

There is evidence suggesting that some patients enact this practice, too. Sharpe (1998) characterises CFS patients as particularly averse to psychological or psychiatric explanations for their illness, and as extremely persistent in holding fixed beliefs concerning their condition. Likewise, analysing interviews with CFS patients, Clark and James (2003) described a kind of anomie coupled with the enforced need to develop a radicalised patient identity that seems to imply a similarly assertive stance.

Practices of pre-emptive defensiveness are not acquired in a social vacuum: they emerge in contexts where some doctors claim that CFS patients exaggerate their symptoms, and that there are discrepancies between their reported symptoms and how they look and behave (Asbring & Narvanen, 2004). These contexts, in turn, may be proximally shaped for doctors by feelings of anxiety in regard to patients' suffering, by their endorsement of scientific procedures to ward off or manage feelings of avoidance, anger and despair, and by feelings of frustration when patients do not respond 'competently' (Fennell, 2003). Fennell also suggests that these feelings instantiate more distal tendencies within medical reasoning to be relatively intolerant of suffering, ambiguity and chronicity, and to beware the economic costs of chronic illness. Studies by Clark and James (2003) and Whitehead (2006) both show that CFS identities were produced in power relations and conflicts between patients, family members, medical professionals and others.

## Implications

This analysis posits a modal CFS sensibility constituted from corporeal practices of somatic monitoring, experiential regulation and pre-emptive defensiveness. These practices organise, manage and respond to extra-emotional feelings of fatigue, pain and weakness, and emotional feelings of fear, anxiety, grief, anger, sadness, guilt and loss, whilst – when successfully enacted – producing and organising further feelings of mastery, self-efficacy and competence. In contingent conjunction with the discursive meanings carried by information about CFS, these corporeal practices constitute feelings of knowing that might range from calm acceptance or grim resignation through to alienation or despair.

Although constituted from related organisations of feeling, discourse and corporeal practice, this sensibility is itself heterogeneous and changeable. It must also be emphasised, again, that not everyone given a CFS diagnosis will acquire this sensibility and that similar sensibilities may arise amongst people given other diagnoses. Moreover, even where present, this sensibility will not be enacted or displayed uniformly. A sensibility is a mutually constitutive organisation of feeling, discourse and practice enacted or interpellated differentially, according to circumstance and situation: a cluster of related potentials or tendencies, not a set of fixed traits that manifest equally in every situation.

The claim that this sensibility might be modal in CFS speaks to the notion that patients are sometimes seen as self-centred complainers who exaggerate their difficulties. Interpersonally, somatic monitoring and experiential regulation could easily appear as self-centredness; similarly, interactional striving to make symptoms count as symptoms, coupled with degrees of pre-emptive defensiveness, might introduce degrees of discomfort and tension on both sides of any encounter.

In encounters with medical professionals this tension might be further exacerbated by doctors' own frequent tendencies to feel anxious, frustrated, despairing, intolerant and wary of CFS patients (Fennell, 2003). The recurrence of such feelings in fact suggests that there is also a modal medical sensibility, one that is constitutive of, and constituted by, the various discourses and practices implicated in the status, training, knowledge and expertise of doctors. Just as CFS sensibilities emerge in relational and material settings that continuously inflect their character, medical sensibilities reflect not only the quasi-omnipotence of an occasional power over life and death, a continuous power over access to services, and a concern with evidence-based practice, but also the more mundane influences of performance assessments, peer reviews, outcome indicators, payment by results and compliance with targets. In a context of severe pressures on health services (produced by a combination of an ageing population, medical advances and ideologically driven spending cuts) these influences might impel a style of 'defensive medicine' that is particularly unhelpful when it encounters CFS patients (Saunders, 2015).

The persistence of negative stereotypes about CFS patients might therefore be understood as the emergent product of a modal CFS sensibility as it interacts with the sensibilities of others, doctors in particular. The CFS stereotype emerges relationally only when that modal sensibility's potentials are activated in interactions with others: and particularly, where its potentials activate contradictory potentials associated with medical training, knowledge and practice. Saunders (2015) describes how doctors in general practice can feel frustrated, helpless, prejudiced towards and set up to fail by CFS patients. Similarly, reflecting on his extensive clinical work in CFS, Ward (2015) describes how patients sometimes made him feel "bruised, confusedly defensive, even angry". Insightfully relating these feelings to medical uncertainty about the condition, Ward suggests that some doctors' own 'ambivalence about ambivalence' might lead them to disavow their difficult feelings about CFS patients. As the next chapter will describe, disavowals of feeling are sometimes associated with hostility and negative judgements, a phenomenon that may help explain why doctors sometimes characterise CFS patients as "demanding, critical, suspicious/sceptical, dissatisfied, pessimistic, too focused on their problems... not being willing to co-operate with the physician, not being willing to accept their situation and being difficult to help" (Åsbring & Närvänen, 2003, p. 718).

In a small way, this analysis also speaks to claims that CFS might be conceptualised as a form of anxious depression. As has been noted, depression itself is a contested classification, one that undergoes frequent mutation: the DSM5, for example, made a significant change to the criteria for major depression by removing the so-called 'bereavement exclusion' (American Psychiatric Association, 2013). Moreover, as with the other so-called functional psychiatric diagnoses, no consistent organic pathology for depression has ever been identified (Cromby, Harper, & Reavey, 2013). It has been noted that the pains and fatigue associated with CFS might well themselves be productive of misery that could be framed as depression. Simultaneously, in interactions with medical professionals and with others, practices of somatic monitoring and experiential regulation could easily come across as expressions of anxiety. Whilst people given a CFS diagnosis might very well appear both miserable and anxious, therefore, this combination could actually be the consequence of their bodily experiences, their uptake of available knowledge, and the practices they consequently enact.[3]

It is important to emphasise that positing the significance of enduring, embodied, socially acquired sensibilities – in CFS, or more generally – does not entail lapsing into either essentialism or naive humanism. A sensibility is not a set of fixed qualities or traits, from which action originates and experience flows. It is, rather, a variable collection of tendencies or potentials, ready to be interpellated in relevant circumstances. Like beliefs, sensibilities endure across situations and are infused with personal significance and meaning; by comparison with beliefs, sensibilities are more implicit and heterogeneous. Moreover, far from sensibilities accreting as structures around unitary, transcendent selves, they are emergent aspects of the dynamic and somewhat autopoietic centres or matrices of acts that constitute our being.

Nonetheless, autopoiesis is always partial because humans are never wholly self-constituting and self-organising: rather, we are always being constituted by powers, influences and processes, many of which we are largely unaware of, and over which, relatively speaking, we have little control (Smail, 1993). Some of these influences and processes are primarily biological, occurring within neural and other systems that operate outwith consciousness; and others are primarily societal and cultural, impelled by largely taken-for-granted aspects of our environments.[4] In this way, sensibilities encounter some of the concerns about consciousness, determinism and agency identified in previous chapters.

Whilst the enduring fatigue and widespread pain associated with CFS might have no consistently identifiable biological cause, this does not mean that they can simply be wished away – any more than can the profound sadness or emotional blankness associated with the diagnosis of depression. Consequently, people with a CFS diagnosis might not so much decide upon a particular sensibility as find themselves effectively *thrown* into one. Rather than reflexively choosing to practice somatic monitoring, for example, CFS patients might come to realise, more or less suddenly – and perhaps only when they encounter information about therapeutic balance – that this is, in fact, what they are already doing. However, far from making this corporeal practice irrational, this eventuality simply illustrates, again, how feeling's primordial constitutive influence sometimes precedes discursive reflection.

# 8
# Maddening

This chapter will explore how feelings contribute to madness. In psychiatry, the bizarre and extreme states of distress experienced by some who receive mental health services are typically described as psychosis, and they are likely to attract a diagnosis of schizophrenia. Like the other functional psychiatric diagnoses, schizophrenia suffers from problems of validity and reliability and – despite over a century of well-funded research using increasingly sophisticated technologies – is not supported by consistent evidence of any biological impairment. When terms such as 'psychosis' and 'schizophrenia' are used uncritically, they covertly import biomedical assumptions into psychology; they are misleading in the degree of certainty they imply about the character of people's distress; and their emphasis on presumed biological vulnerabilities can cause relevant relational, social and material influences to be downplayed. For these reasons, some psychologists increasingly use the ordinary language term 'madness' to index the forms of distress that psychiatrists call psychosis and schizophrenia (e.g. Bentall, 2003). Nevertheless, to avoid misrepresentation, 'psychosis' and 'schizophrenia' will still be used in this chapter when referring to or quoting from others who have deployed these terms.

The non-medical emphasis is warranted by a series of influential recent works, many from within UK clinical psychology, which provide evidence and analysis demonstrating the limitations of psychiatric disease concepts and, simultaneously, highlight the utility and richness of consistently psychological accounts. In a series of important books, Smail (1984, 1987, 1993, 2005) showed how combinations of toxic social and material forces produce clinical distress. These forces are mediated through families and by others with whom we have proximal relationships – relationships which may sometimes exert unhelpful influences of their own, particularly where trauma and abuse are present (Johnstone, 2000; Harrop & Trower, 2003; Read et al., 2005). Focusing specifically on madness, Boyle (2002) showed that the methodology by which the concept of schizophrenia was derived was inadequate and that later work refining it has not addressed these shortcomings. Subsequent work by Bentall (2003) and colleagues has both supplied psychological models of madness (and other forms of distress) and demonstrated the efficacy of psychological interventions. These clinical psychological works are informed by two other important contemporary developments. First, the service user movement, particularly the UK 'Hearing Voices Network' which was inspired by the work of Romme and Escher (1993) to develop peer support groups of voice-hearers who collectively manage their experiences in non-stigmatising ways. Second, the Critical Psychiatry Network (Double, 2006), a group of psychiatrists who are challenging their discipline's orthodoxies with respect to issues such as how psychiatric medication functions (Moncrieff, 2008) or what diagnoses such as attention-deficit hyperactivity disorder (ADHD) actually index (Timimi & Taylor, 2004). Together, these three movements are beginning to provide an effective alternative to the individualising, reductionist and stigmatising biological disease notions which, despite a distinct lack of supporting evidence, psychiatry still promotes.

Whilst this chapter will consider madness in general, the latter half which explores social and material influences will focus more specifically on paranoia: experiences of perceiving and relating to others that are characterised by suspicion, mistrust or hostility. Paranoia is a common everyday experience, but amongst those receiving mental health services it is frequently characterised by complex, self-insulating belief systems, distorted perceptions and significant emotional distress.

## Relational feeling and madness

> Over the next few days, Jenny slowly lost her hold on reality. The heavy sedative effects [of psychiatric drugs] were accompanied by a restlessness that kept her constantly on the move up and down the ward, muttering under her breath and occasionally pulling up her nightdress to show the nurses her supposedly too-large hips. From time to time she had outbursts...she threw food and plates around, tried to escape from the ward, swore at the doctors, slammed doors, and hurled herself to the floor...At other times, it seemed as though her previous worries were all appearing in a distorted form. For instance, she told the staff that Prince Charming had spoken to

her from the television ... that she was a film star, and then that she was pregnant. Once she asked anxiously if she had killed her family, and then told one of the doctors 'I'm only three years old'.

(Johnstone, 2000, p. 69)

Lucy Johnstone provides a detailed analysis showing how a combination of emotional sensitivity and overwrought, conflicted family dynamics together produced a fraught situation which culminated in Jenny's being given a diagnosis of schizophrenia. The short excerpt above describes Jenny in the days immediately following her diagnosis and hospitalisation and details some of the beliefs she proclaimed at this time. Johnstone's analysis sensitively renders these seemingly bizarre beliefs sensible, clearly showing how they relate directly to Jenny's relational and material circumstances.

Jenny grew up in a household with a somewhat distant father and a relatively protective mother. Her parents' relationship had irretrievably broken down early in Jenny's life, but its appearance was stonily and ungenerously maintained because of social conventions. At school Jenny had always struggled to make friends, and when she progressed to college her difficulties continued – compounded now by tentative, barely articulable sexual desires, coupled with a self-perception that she was unattractive because she had big hips and freckles. After a lengthy period of sullen withdrawal, social isolation and arguing with her parents, with the friendly encouragement of a sympathetic GP Jenny began to make small efforts to gain independence and maybe realise her fantasy of becoming a film star: she began to contact old friends, go out more and diet. But these attempts to develop her life outside the home only produced more anxiety and conflict within it, because they provoked her mother's fears that Jenny would move away and, in so doing, both abandon her and expose the sham of her marriage. Impelled by these conflicting intentions, the seething tension in Jenny's home erupted into furious conflict, with Jenny screaming that her mother wanted to keep her like a child and her mother screaming back that Jenny was mad and needed to be locked up. A locum doctor called out by Jenny's mother was unable to resolve the arguing, but was alarmed by Jenny's unusual remarks ('I can fly out of here any time I want, you know ... I know the GP is really married to me, I know everything') so called a psychiatrist and duty social worker. A provisional diagnosis of schizophrenia was made and Jenny was hospitalised.

Johnstone uses Jenny's story to show how family dynamics can contribute to distress, suggesting that conflicts are sometimes resolved by artificially locating the problem solely within one family member and diagnosing her or him as 'ill'.[1] Here, Jenny's story will be considered in a parallel fashion, to demonstrate the role of feelings in constituting distress and producing unusual beliefs. In Johnstone's account, many strong feelings run through Jenny's story. The home was 'tense', and Jenny's mother continually expressed 'bitterness and resentment' toward her father. When Jenny first became 'withdrawn' and the GP was called out, he decided she was 'confused' and 'unhappy'. Jenny blamed her parents for having created an atmosphere that would 'make anyone miserable', although her ambition to become a film star gave her 'hope'. The GP's support initially triggered positive changes for Jenny, who began going out more, although the thought of sex and relationships was 'terrifying' and provoked 'bitter' memories of being teased and ridiculed. One day Jenny came to the surgery alone, 'cheerful and confident', having spent some of her savings on clothes and planned a night out. But the next day the GP received a 'frantic' call from Jenny's mother, saying that Jenny was going mad; despite reassurances that this was unlikely the calls continued so he visited Jenny's home a day later. He found Jenny 'openly angry', 'furious' with her mother, who was 'yelling back' and calling Jenny crazy. The GP tried to calm the situation but feelings were 'running too high'. Later, when the locum arrived, Jenny was 'extremely agitated' and her mother still 'yelling'. The two had a 'furious screaming match', after which the locum called for psychiatric assistance. After being diagnosed Jenny struggled 'desperately' and on admission to the ward 'angrily' refused to be examined so was forcibly sedated.

Johnstone (2000, pp. 73–74) suggests that, whilst most people sometimes speak in metaphors, people in the extremes of distress "take the process a stage further and start living their metaphors instead" and this is what psychiatry takes to be their 'delusional beliefs'. Her account shows how Jenny's superficially bizarre beliefs are in fact sensible in the context of her circumstances. It also accords with the notion that beliefs are organisations of feeling contingently allied to discourse, since each of Jenny's beliefs can be related to one or more of the conflicting feelings that came to dominate her life in the days before and after her hospitalisation. For example, Jenny's claim that 'I'm only three years old' relates to her deep and enduring feelings of helplessness and disempowerment: in relation to her mother and father, in her seeming inability to change her life for the better, and in the hospital ward where she was forcibly detained. Other beliefs (being pregnant, having killed her family) are imbued with fear and anxiety, relating to Jenny's terror about sexual relations and her reasonable anxiety that, however the current crisis is resolved, her family will never be the same again. More poignantly, Jenny's beliefs that 'Prince Charming' had spoken to her and that she would one day be a film star reflect her thwarted desires to escape the miserable family home and make a better life.

In these ways, the notion of belief as an organisation of feeling contingently allied to discourse is broadly consonant with Jenny's story. However, it can also be used to extend our understanding of Jenny's situation by considering what actually happens in this move from metaphor ('I feel like a little child') to belief ('I'm only three years old'). If beliefs are, most fundamentally, organisations of feeling, such a move must speak to the sheer intensity, depth and persistence of Jenny's feelings of helplessness. Similarly, the unconventional way these feelings inflect Jenny's discourse – such that her beliefs are readily taken as delusional – suggests something of their uncontrollability, the way in which her feelings are so powerful and readily present that their unbidden influence might surge forth at any time. What needs to be explained, then, is how Jenny's feelings might have both attained such a pitch and persisted for such a lengthy period: for this, the notion of *feeling traps* can be used.

### Feeling traps and 'florid' states

The concept of feeling traps was first described by Lewis (1971), on the basis of her analysis of a large corpus of psychotherapeutic interactions. Recently, it has been popularised by Scheff (2003) who, like Lewis, especially emphasises the importance of shame (which he treats as the core term within a 'family' of related feelings such as embarrassment and self-consciousness).[2] Feeling traps occur when circumstances lead feelings to form self-perpetuating loops with others: this causes these feelings to be intensified, sustained over time and generalised across social situations. This is especially likely when feelings are 'bypassed' or 'disavowed': when a person does not, or is not able, to acknowledge and act upon a feeling, instead trying to act as though it were not present. Lewis found that in her data shame was almost never mentioned or acknowledged. However, when clients described situations where shame might reasonably be expected to be relevant, but did not acknowledge its presence, in every case their subsequent talk was inflected with anger: a shame/anger feeling trap. In recent years feeling traps have been invoked within explanations of phenomena as varied as conflicts between (groups of) academics (Brooks-Bouson, 2005), post-traumatic symptoms (Herman, 2007), false-consciousness of social class (Scheff & Mahlendorf, 1988), dominant American attitudes toward 'poor white trash' (Brooks-Bouson, 2001), atrocities (Vetlesen, 2011), multiple killing (Scheff, 2011), bullying (Martocci, 2015) and riots (Ray, 2014).

For example, Scheff (2003) uses biographies of Adolf Hitler to show how his early childhood was characterised by an ongoing feeling trap where anger, humiliation and abuse by his father was paralleled by adoration and love from his mother. Despite continually telling the young Adolf that she loved him, his mother failed to protect him from his father and never acknowledged the abuse that occurred. Hitler grew up within an affective dynamic which predisposed him to feel rage and shame at the treatment meted out by his father, yet simultaneously to deny or ignore these feelings because they were not validated or acknowledged, by his mother or anyone else. Scheff proposes that many elements of Hitler's later comportment and behaviour – his piercing stare, obsessive character, temper tantrums, anger and continual preoccupation with pride – derive from his early socialisation within this feeling trap, which endowed him with strong propensities toward shame whilst simultaneously training him to disavow this feeling. Consequently, Hitler veered between two different but equally shame-oriented ways of being in the world, according to circumstance. He sometimes managed a complete disavowal of his shame, evidenced by corporeal practices of rapid, high pressure speech, an aggressive domineering manner and a piercing stare, coupled with an obsessive narrative style where tropes and invocations of pride frequently figured. But in other circumstances, and even long after he became Chancellor, Hitler's demeanour was characterised by fawning obsequiousness, excessive humility, and consistent talk of his low status and profound lack of worth.[3]

Whilst Scheff is clear that Hitler's socialisation only explains aspects of his character and ways of relating, and not his politics or ideology, he does draw parallels between Hitler's obsessive preoccupations with shame and pride and the prevailing mood amongst the German people, which was often characterised by resentment and humiliation following the punitive settlement imposed under the Treaty of Versailles at the end of the First World War. Scheff's claim is not that the economics and geopolitics of this situation can be reduced to feelings, simply that there was a resonance between this cultural mood and Hitler's personal affective dynamics. Hitler's speeches were, from a logical point of view "disasters" and his political program "disorganised, vague, and silent on key issues" (op. cit., p. 746), but Hitler nevertheless inspired fanatical loyalty because his propensities toward shame and pride mirrored and channelled those of the wider culture:

Hitler's obsession with restoring his lost pride and that of his nation was the key to his vast appeal to his public and his followers, because they were suffering from exactly the same shame as he was, in the aftermath of their defeat in WW1 and their ensuring humiliations.

(Scheff, 2003, p. 746)

Scheff also touches upon the relevance of feeling traps to distress when his reading of biographies of Hitler leads him to conclude that:

Hitler's personality was bizarre to the point of madness. His delusions, phobias, sadism, sexual aberrations and utter isolation are well documented. All of the biographies clearly show manifold symptoms of severe mental illness.

(op. cit.)

It must nevertheless be emphasised that feeling traps are not necessarily profoundly damaging. Scheff also mentions the relatively innocuous example of compulsive blushing, which occurs when feelings of anxiety and embarrassment magnify and sustain each other. Being in love and having that love reciprocated is also a feeling trap – ostensibly an entirely benign situation, despite its occasional description as a form of mental illness not recognised in any diagnostic manual (Sutherland, 1996). Like other constituents of experience, those which produce feeling traps intersect contingently with others that sometimes moderate, and sometimes amplify, their effects: their mere presence need not signify difficulties. However, when persistent combinations of circumstance effectively 'lock' individuals into enduring, complex mixtures of potent feelings, particularly shame – and especially when one or more of these feelings are disavowed or bypassed – the consequences can be toxic.

Developing this argument in relation to distress, Scheff (2013) proposes that feeling traps can induce spirals that are recursive without intrinsic limit, for example in shame/shame sequences: being ashamed that you are ashamed. These spirals can be sustained virtually (in relation to the imagined or anticipated evaluations of others) and actually, in lived social relations. Scheff emphasises feeling traps of shame/shame, shame/anger and shame/fear, suggesting that these mixtures are likely to constitute the experiences associated with a diagnosis of depression, and to sometimes precipitate interpersonal violence. Other mixtures of feelings might nevertheless be implicated in distress: in Jenny's case, these mixtures potentially encompassed shame, resentment, frustration, bitterness, sexual desire, affection, helplessness, anxiety, fear, anger and hope. Many of these feelings have potentials to sustain and magnify others, to be interpellated in response to others, to be enacted as 'masks', diversions or disavowals for others, or to arise as (over-)compensations for others. Sexual desire, for example, might variously interpellate shame, excitement, hope, anxiety, love or affection. Helplessness might call out resentment, bitterness, fear or anxiety, but also sadness and longing. And, whilst humiliation and shame most readily interpellate anger, the 'Fifty Shades of Grey' phenomenon unhelpfully eroticises male domination but also reveals more complex possibilities for the uptake and effects of these feelings (Downing, 2012), possibilities also suggested by some psychotherapeutic evidence (Barker, Iantaffi, & Gupta, 2007; Lindemann, 2011).

Illustrating some of these kinds of complexities, Johnstone shows that, whilst Jenny's mother feared Jenny leaving home, Jenny herself was frightened to leave even though she desperately wanted to do so. Jenny feared abandonment at the same time as she yearned to be independent; felt angry at her parents whilst also needing their love; felt helpless, even as she seethed with anger and resentment. Aspects of Jenny's behaviour (her shyness, her overly critical stance towards her own body, throwing herself on the hospital floor) suggest that she also experienced strong feelings of insecurity, shame or self-loathing, feelings she sometimes disavowed and sometimes enacted graphically. Simultaneously, Jenny's mother was also gripped by mixtures of powerful feelings, and these provoked, reinforced and complemented those her daughter was experiencing.

Experience is constituted from multiple, parallel processes that always include a flux of feelings prompted by *material* circumstances. Many of these feelings are interpellated more or less fleetingly and temporarily by aspects of the material environment: the comfort of our chair, the temperature, the humidity, how hungry or thirsty we are and so on. But there are also more profound material influences that operate at different speeds to produce regimes of feeling that locate experience much more subtly and continuously within the local material ecology. These influences are primarily regulated by processes of biological entrainment. Through entrainment, the cycles that govern biological activity – known as circadian clocks, or biorhythms – synchronise with location-specific diurnal cycles (Roenneberg et al., 2007) by using ecological features such as light intensity, temperature and resource availability that act as 'zeitgebers' or time signals. Humans have multiple circadian clocks: there is a centrally organising rhythm enabled by a brain region just above the optical chiasm, but there are also others – the liver, for example, has its own rhythm that, in rats, can be entrained by feeding patterns (Stokkan et al., 2001). In general, these rhythms align feelings of hunger, sleepiness, attentiveness and acuity with local cycles of day and night and with typical patterns of activity, rest and sleep. However, we only tend to remark upon or notice these various feelings on the typically rare occasions when they suddenly become starkly asynchronous with activity: for example, when the abrupt dys-entrainment of jet lag makes them unpleasantly prominent.[4]

Experiences of continuity can also arise from socially interpellated feelings. Chapter 3 described how somatic repertoires associated with sociological distinctions such as class and gender can produce broadly consistent organisations of feeling which then get cross-cut with more local influences such as those induced within specific work or leisure situations. Indeed, the great majority of feelings tend to smoothly align, each with the other, just as they mostly 'run together' with both the signs and symbols we encounter (Ruthrof, 1997) and the 'synaesthetically predictable' (Merleau-Ponty, 2002) textures of the surfaces and objects we occupy and use.

In short, whether induced materially or interpellated socially, feelings constitute experiences of fluidity and change *and* experiences of continuity and stability. Jenny's story illustrates how relational influences can produce powerful mixtures of feelings that are disruptive both because they are so intense and because they are disjunctive with current circumstance. Since feeling traps tend to sustain, intensify and generalise mixtures of feeling, they have considerable potential to produce strong feelings that are disjunctive in this way: this frequently causes them to be disavowed, which in turn can cause them to be further magnified and sustained.

This led Dave Harper and I (Cromby & Harper, 2009) to suggest that when feeling traps get sufficiently prolonged, they may induce such highly aroused states that self-reinforcing mixtures of feeling surge forth unpredictably. Mixtures of overt and bypassed relational feelings temporarily overwhelm the feelings constitutive of continuity and stability, and so dominate perceptions and discourse. We argued that this is how so-called 'florid' states are produced: but rather than being the outcome of faulty brains, these states are relationally generated within the embodied dialectical exchanges between perception, discourse, feeling and circumstance.

Once they have occurred, florid states bear their own significant meanings. Bodily, they may act as tipping points, momentous occasions when the apparent security and solidity of the world, usually given effortlessly by our embodied engagements within it, is suddenly, shockingly, revealed as a somewhat fragile achievement. In this way, what Laing (1960) called 'ontological insecurity' might be just as much an effect as a cause of distress, its experience serving to endow moments of floridity with greatly increased salience. Socially, they may be stigmatising, devaluing and frightening because of their widely recognised associations with pathology, illness and deviance, associations frequently emphasised by the trauma of hospitalisation and (sometimes forcible) treatment, experiences likely to themselves engender feelings of panic and loss of control (Morrison, Frame, & Larkin, 2003).

This seems to be what happened for Jenny, whose enduring mixtures of conflicting feelings, locked into place by her actual position of relative powerlessness, became so intense and unpredictable that, even before her hospitalisation, they began impelling her talk in unconventional ways ('I can fly out of here any time I want. I know the GP is really married to me . . . '). Her diagnosis and subsequent hospitalisation, far from alleviating these powerful feelings, added further feelings of shock and fear. Consequently, far from abating, Jenny's complex mixtures of extreme feelings began shaping her perceptions to the extent that once she was on the ward she heard 'Prince Charming' speaking from the television.

It is at this kind of point, where people see and hear things not within the consensual reality of others, that the idea of distress as biological disease might seem to have its strongest pull. Hallucinations are often clearly dysfunctional, outwith 'normal' perceptual experience, and disturbing for those who experience them; attributing them to organic disease might therefore seem plausible. Nevertheless, in everyday life it is also widely recognised that feeling has a continuous influence upon perception. Consider the rose-coloured spectacles of people newly in love, or the flat, colourless world of the deeply miserable. These descriptions are not just figures of speech: they are also lay recognitions that the felt, dynamic body helps generate the experienced world. In this regard, Langer (1967, 1982) highlights the importance of a kind of 'physiognomic seeing' wherein objects and places are perceived in terms of their felt values and affordances as much as their objective characteristics. Meanings and perceptions are intimately bound up with bodily processes and activities, so that the world we occupy is one always already suffused by feelings that give it meaning:

> The light of a candle changes its appearance for a child when, after a burn, it stops attracting the child's hand and becomes quite literally

repulsive. Vision is already inhabited by a meaning (*sens*) which gives it a function in the spectacle of the world and in our existence.

(Merleau-Ponty, 2002, p. 60)

Hence people who have lost a loved one frequently 'see' her or him in the faces of passers-by, and people expecting a baby 'see' pregnant women everywhere. Similarly, experimental evidence demonstrates that poor people 'see' high value bank notes as larger (Bruner & Goodman, 1947), people afraid of spiders locate them in an array more readily than other people (Ohman, Flykt, & Esteves, 2001), and (in Anglo-American cultures, though not elsewhere – Lee, 2001) people with eating disorders 'see' their own bodies as larger than they actually are (Jansen et al., 2006). And in Jenny's case, perhaps, her thwarted and disavowed desires reached such a pitch that they temporarily over-whelmed the socially and materially produced feelings rooting her in the shared consensual world, so that she 'heard' Prince Charming speaking to her.

## Societal feeling and paranoia

Whilst relational feelings can be constitutive of madness, there are also well-established associations between madness and adverse social and material conditions (social inequality, deprivation, marginalisation and abuse) and a range of social structural influences including gender, ethnicity and urban living.

Evidence that madness is significantly more common amongst poorer, disadvantaged and marginalised people goes back many decades (e.g. Tietze et al., 1941), and by the mid-1970s this was so consistent that Kohn (1976, p. 177) concluded that

> [t]here have been more than 50 studies of the relationship between social class and rates of schizophrenia. Almost without exception, these studies have shown that schizophrenia occurs most frequently at the lowest social class levels of urban society. The evidence comes from research in Canada, Denmark, Finland, Great Britain, Norway, Sweden, Taiwan, and the United States – an unusually large num-ber of countries and cultures for establishing the generality of any relationship in social science.

These associations hold today: a longitudinal case-control study by Harrison, Gunnell, Glazebrook, Page and Kwiecinski (2001) showed that being born in a deprived area to parents who are in unskilled labour or unemployed increased the adult risk of a schizophrenia diagnosis more than eight times; a birth-cohort study with a larger sample of nearly 72,000 people (Werner, Malaspina, & Rabinowitz, 2007) found similar associations, albeit at lower levels. Conversely, a study using the Danish national register found little evidence for the influence of parental SES, but reconfirmed the linking between diagnoses of schizophrenia and contemporaneous unemployment, low educational attainment and lower income (Byrne et al., 2004). Independently of income inequality, there is a relationship between minority ethnic status and schizophrenia, with black and Asian people in the UK 50% more likely to be given diagnoses than white people (King et al., 1994). Genetic explanations for this imbalance have been suggested, but evidence here is both unconvincing (Sharpley, Hutchinson, & Murray, 2001) and rendered implausible by evidence showing that the prevalence of schizophrenia diagnoses is higher among black people living in majority white areas (Boydell et al., 2001).

These societal or sociological associations also need to be explained, and for this it will be useful to consider those modes of mad experience we call 'paranoia'. Studies have shown that paranoia is associated with immigration and low socio-economic status (Kendler, 1982), refugee status (Westermeyer, 1989), victimisation and stressful life events (Johns et al., 2004). There is also some evidence associating madness in clinical populations and paranoia in the general population (Johns et al., 2004) to maleness: in their study controlling for the confounding effects of urbanicity and migration, Scully et al. (2002) found that paranoid and other core schizophrenia diagnoses were 7.5 times more likely to be given to men than women.

Three psychological models of paranoia have recently dominated the literature and each, in different ways, places considerable emphasis on emotion and feeling. The attributional model (Bentall et al., 2001) proposes that paranoid delusions are causal attributions made as part of dysfunctional or ineffective attempts to regulate, conceal or avoid feelings of low self-esteem: they therefore serve a defensive function. By contrast, Freeman, Garety, Kuipers, Fowler and Bebbington (2002) propose that paranoid delusions directly reflect individual emotional states, particularly anxiety, and that their content is therefore congruent with individual's current emotional status. Finally, Trower and Chadwick (1995) identify two types of paranoia, both serving a different defensive function. The most prevalent 'poor me' paranoia defends an insecure self from abandonment and lack of recognition, resulting in grandiose delusions where anger is prominent. The less prevalent 'bad me' paranoia defends an alienated self from intrusion, entrapment and domination, resulting in persecutory delusions, shame and misery. All three models have attracted considerable interest from clinicians and researchers. Whilst they are frequently seen as competing or mutually exclusive, they might equally be seen as illuminating different aspects, characteristics or forms of these puzzling experiences.

At the same time, these models have shortcomings that limit their explanatory power. First, all three orient toward cognitive psychology, and to that extent invoke a relatively stark distinction between cognition and affect or emotion and thought.[5] Second, they invoke a relatively individual and static conception of emotion, where it is both differentiated from thought and typically arises either episodically and discretely or continuously and uniformly.[6] Third, and most importantly for the present argument, all three models are relatively blind to social and material influence, and each posits dynamics of cognition and emotion that seemingly arise with little specific reference to circumstances. For example, Freeman et al. (2002) briefly mention social isolation with respect to persecutory delusions, but only in association with supposed individual tendencies to "be secretive or mistrustful...or believe that personal matters should not be discussed with others" (Freeman et al., 2002, p. 336). Similarly, they conclude a lengthy list of internal, cognitive processes that may help to maintain delusions with the cursory statement that: "Finally, the person's interactions with others may become disturbed. The person may act upon their delusions in a way that elicits hostility or isolation" (Freeman et al., 2002, p. 338). In such ways, relational influence is simultaneously acknowledged and constrained, relegated to a subordinate position where cognitive processes have causal primacy. Similarly, Bentall and Kaney (2005) discuss the attribution-self representation cycle in ways that rhetorically downplay relational influence, deploying a cognitive language of 'pessimistic attributions' and 'changing beliefs about the self' that seemingly arise and interact with little reference to circumstance or situation. And although Trower and Chadwick (1995) endorse social constructionist notions of self their account is almost entirely relational and individual, with only occasional undeveloped references to 'the other' and 'public/private distinctions' to vaguely suggest the wider material and social world wherein these relationships and experiences occur.

These models do not adequately acknowledge that what we say about ourselves and our world influences how others respond to us, and this in turn influences how we think and feel. Social, relational and material influences are frequently translated into internal, mechanical ones, or described without reference to the material circumstances and social structures by which they are mediated. More generally, relationality is obfuscated through psychology's preoccupation with the individual and relative neglect of the responses of others involved in interaction (Georgaca, 2004; Harper, 2004), a stance that ignores how people experiencing paranoia may be subject to reactions of others that could be viewed as conspiratorial (Lemert, 1962). Whilst versions of the dynamics they posit might well occur, the models are demonstrably incomplete because these dynamics never operate independently of social influence. Consequently, even for these *psychological* models, clinical paranoia tends to appear as the bizarre, dysfunctional behaviour of deviant individuals – rather than an understandable response to toxic combinations of social and material circumstances, relational trajectories and life events.

## Paranoia: A social account

> Mark: He's a guy that lives around – he's a criminal, he's a murderer, he's a thief, he's a liar, he's a dud, he's a copy, he's a clown person. He's a copy of myself as impersonates me and all my stuff and he's a clown person, changes different appearances. It's hard to explain but the FBI are very advanced in technology, goes to the moon and you know Mars and all them places you know so it's very advanced technology.
>
> (Cromby, Harper, & Sutton, 2006)

In the three clinical psychological models, paranoia narratives such as Mark's can either be defensive of self or expressive of anxiety. Even where they are understood as expressive, however, it will always be the case that they express anxiety *in a particular way*: Mark's story, for example, renders anxiety more reasonable through the accumulation of detail. It also demonstrates how paranoia narratives frequently position the speaker as relatively important or powerful, or in possession of arcane or specialist knowledge which – if true – might raise their social status. This function is likely to be especially salient for most who enter the realm of treatment and diagnosis, because the stigmatising associations of 'mental illness', and associated discriminatory social practices (e.g. exclusion from employment), are widely recognised (Sayce, 1998). This may be especially so during interactions with professionals, where self-presentations are not only interactionally relevant but may have additional significance because of their possible influence upon treatment or related decisions. In this context paranoia narratives (like all narratives) will be oriented towards the situated demands of social interaction: consequently, accounts imbued with some degree of self-aggrandisement, and with the interactional consequence (if believed) of raising their author's apparent status, are often prevalent: Trower and Chadwick (1995) describe these narratives as 'grandiose'.

Whilst the specific feelings that constitute paranoia for any given individual will vary, researchers consistently identify some feelings that are more prevalent than others. It is widely accepted that fear or anxiety is common, as are feelings of shame, embarrassment or diminished self-worth. In addition, and although it figures less often (Combs, Michael, & Penn, 2006) there is reason to suppose that feelings of anger are often significant. First, narrative accounts presume the hostility of others and so, by relational reciprocity, suggest at least the possibility of anger on the part of those generating them (as in Trower and Chadwick's model of 'poor me' paranoia, which similarly predicts the presence of anger). Second, Lewis (1971) found that bypassed shame was frequently followed by feelings of anger, and paranoia narratives display evidence of bypassed shame (rapid speech and obsessive preoccupation). Third, a small minority of people who experience paranoia do become angry and violent – typically toward people they know, but sometimes towards strangers.

Feelings such as fear, shame and anger are always in continual, relational exchange with ongoing social interaction. One consequence of this is that paranoia ebbs and flows, according to changing relational and material circumstances (Garety, 1985). Another is that the mixtures of (for example) fear, shame and anger that constitute paranoia can impel discursive and corporeal practices which themselves increase social isolation, marginalisation and stigmatisation. Individuals who persistently talk and act in paranoid ways are likely to encounter disbelief, rejection and mistrust from others, responses which may generate additional feelings of fear, shame and anger – feelings which, in turn, may further intensify their paranoia. In this way individuals may acquire habits of feeling that then operate pre-reflectively, structuring perceptions and activity in ways that seem simply given.

Simultaneously, the responses of others may also assume habitual characteristics, perhaps of being wary about the person or vigilant about one's social contact with them. Unhelpful trajectories of relating can ensue: feelingful modes of experience characterised by mixtures of fear, shame and anger can propitiate corporeal practices and discursive constructions that generate yet more of these feelings. The interpenetration, flow and exchange of relational dynamics and felt experience can mean that perceptions repeatedly get structured by low-level mixtures of anger, shame and fear; their interpenetration can reach such a pitch that reality momentarily becomes wholly terrifying, hostile or shaming; and both of these can occur, episodically or alternately.

Running through these social and relational processes may also be what Langer characterises as a deep human need to make assertions. In her analysis "assertion is one of the primary acts of mind" (Langer, 1982, p. 20), because in the process of declaring that events have such-and-such a character we also affirm our own disposition, ability and worth. The emotional value and felt import attached to relatively dogmatic statements derives in considerable part from their parallel utility in affirming the integrity and value of the self: "It is in making assertions about the world as a whole that the mind affirms itself as a whole" (op. cit., p. 25). This affirmative function may therefore become especially important in situations of relational turmoil and societal impotence, precisely because the felt needed for such affirmation is greater whilst other available sources to exercise power and elevate relative status are simultaneously not available.

Another important consideration is that emotional feelings which persist can eventually diminish. Frijda (1988, p. 353) describes this as "the law of habituation: Continued pleasures wear off; continued hardships lose their poignancy." Habituation has been studied using behavioural measures such as the orienting response, and in relation to topics such as phobic exposure and pain from noxious stimuli. With the advent of brain imaging researchers have studied habituation at the neural level, for example demonstrating differential patterns of neural habituation to emotional faces between amygdala and prefrontal cortex (Wright et al., 2001) and showing that habituation to affective faces occurs within a right-hemisphere neural network containing areas implicated in facial recognition (Feinstein et al., 2002). Whilst there nevertheless seem to be few studies of emotional or *phenomenological* habituation, Fridja contends that his 'law' is copiously supported by experience:

> Daily life offers ample illustrations again, partly consoling ones, partly saddening ones. The pains of loss of love abate with time, but love itself gradually loses its magic. Continued exposure to inhumanities blunts both suffering and moral discernment.
>
> (Fridja, 1988, p. 353)

These examples can be supplemented by others more closely associated with distress. The recently bereaved may appear profoundly sad whilst saying only that they don't feel anything, or that they feel 'numb' (Bennett & Vidal-Hall, 2000). Similarly, people traumatised following an accident may appear intensely agitated whilst denying that they actually feel anxiety. So whilst the bodily and neural systems that enable emotional feelings might be active, people's *experience* of emotional feeling can habituate and anxiety (for example) become unfelt anxiety.[7]

Phenomenological habituation to emotional feelings may help account for the persistence of the psychiatric distinction between the 'cognitive' disorder of schizophrenia and 'affective' bipolar disorder (although other differences, for example in articulacy and socioeconomic status, no doubt also contribute). It might also feed into, and be sustained by, social and relational pressures to disavow certain feelings. On the one hand, it may facilitate disavowal by generating the experiential illusion that certain feelings really have been neutralised. On the other, it may make their eruptions back into experience more likely, less explicable, and correspondingly more difficult to manage or account for.

Especially when habituation occurs, feeling traps structured by mixtures of fear, shame, anger and other feelings may generate highly aroused or florid paranoid states. Whilst most will avoid such experiences, everyone has perhaps at least glimpsed the potency and strangeness that characterise moments where the world itself, albeit fleetingly, takes on the character of their most precious desires, hopes and fears. When this happens to people their talk may become more rapid (so called 'pressure of speech') as they strive to bypass or disavow toxic feelings. Their narratives may become disjointed as they struggle to interpret their multiple, fluctuating feelings and the fragments of meaning attached to them – so-called 'thought disorder'. Likewise, their logic – reflecting the complex, mobile, partially unspeakable mix of feelings within it – may defy some everyday conventions whilst entirely according with others, and indeed whilst reflecting in important ways the events, people and circumstances with which they are currently preoccupied. They may also adopt particular corporeal practices such as being highly active, restless, walking, keeping busy and seeking expansive, open spaces (McGrath & Reavey, 2015).

Hence, Mark's talk is rapid, beginning with a repetitive list of derogatory assessments emphasising the unusual trope of the 'clown person', the details of which construct a threatening figure whose influence would surely cause anyone concern. Yet the overall structure is disjointed: whilst Mark's narrative is presented as though it were a logical argument, the putative connections between 'clown person', space travel and the FBI are not explained. His narrative invokes a sense of powerful forces and mysterious technologies, a feeling of connection and power, whilst simultaneously constructing his 'clown person' antagonist as someone to be feared yet perhaps also laughed at: a construction that simultaneously enacts anxiety *and* defensively asserts his own status by comparison. Mark's narrative, then, fulfils an immediate relational function where it both manages and enacts patterns of feeling whilst simultaneously explaining and justifying them.

Developing a comprehensively social account requires explicit consideration of how feelings and narratives are societal, as well as relational. Whilst Mark's narrative serves an immediate interpersonal function, in managing his status it simultaneously orients toward institutional hierarchies extending beyond the immediate realm of its speaking. Relationships and interactions follow social codes, invoke culturally normative morals and values, are worked up through available and legitimated discourses, involve accepted subject positions (associated with gender, ethnicity, age and so on), and are oriented toward objects and institutions in the shared social world. It follows that the relational dynamics of feeling traps are frequently inflected by socially significant distinctions such as gender and ethnicity.

One problem of much research into paranoia is its focus on abstract, de-contextualised notions of paranoia, rather than the paranoia that might be experienced by a person of, say, a certain gender, age, class or ethnicity. When forms of difference are investigated, such research typically seeks gross differences between groups, rather than exploring subtle, nuanced variation in the meaning and signification of actual concrete experiences. It is nevertheless possible that the empirical associations between maleness and paranoia might in part be due to patterns of male socialisation and their associated relational expectations of strength and the ability to protect, provide, care for and watch over others. Similarly racism, in the gross form of physical assaults, verbal abuse, prejudice and discrimination, as well as more subtle, continuous everyday minor omissions and slights, might partially explain the association between minority ethnic status and paranoia (Chakraborty & McKenzie, 2002). In a gendered, racially discriminatory society, being both male and non-white is likely to be associated with relational dynamics characterised on the one hand by suspicion, mistrust, vigilance, apprehension, and anxiety, and on the other by strong imperatives to deny and disavow these feelings in order to appear proud, competent, confident and strong. Moreover, normative expectations around gender roles, racial prejudice and discrimination may mean that similar feelings, discourses and practices, including those associated with paranoia, signify differently: hence, fear and anxiety associated with threatening city-centre environments can get configured as either 'streetwise' or 'silly', depending on gender (Edley & Wetherell, 1995).

Feeling traps incorporate their extra-verbal, material situation just as much as they do the interpersonal or psychological dimensions of those relating (cf. Brown & Stenner, 2009). Consequently, by jointly examining relational dynamics, social structures and material elements, an explanation for the empirical association between paranoia and social inequality might be constructed. It must nevertheless be emphasised that social inequality is not uniform, does not impact upon people uniformly, and is not responded to uniformly. The great variety of dynamically interacting cultural forms, corporeal practices, lines of power, spatial and material organisations and temporal shifts that constitute experience mean there are always degrees of contingency and chaos, and unexpected outcomes can always emerge (Cromby, Harper, & Reavey, 2013). So, just as not all experiences of male socialisation or racist social relations produce paranoia, paranoia is neither confined to disadvantaged groups, nor ubiquitous amongst them. Nevertheless, three sets of reasons why paranoia will be more prevalent in conditions of social inequality can be identified.

First, some kinds of relational dynamics will be more prevalent or significant in conditions of persistent social inequality. Charlesworth's (1999) ethnographic study shows how the exigencies of dealing with low status, low pay, long hours, job insecurity or unemployment are copiously productive of anxiety, misery, despair, anger and shame.[8] Simultaneously, material demands to persist in coping with both these feelings and the circumstances that interpellated them may encourage tendencies to disavowal or bypassing. These feelings and their consequences can impact negatively upon family life and relationships, imbuing them with a toxic character derived from the wider social realm. Accordingly, it is to be expected that some people will favour styles of corporeal practice that are relatively hostile, controlling and emotionally guarded, and that these people will often be men because these styles resonate with already-dominant gender stereotypes.

Whilst functional in some circumstances these ways of relating can also have negative consequences – especially, perhaps, when they inhabit parenting. Relatedly, people may have less time and ability to enact discursive and corporeal practices that bestow upon others affection, love and reassurance that could somewhat insulate against the negative feelings their social world inculcates. Additionally, shaming and hostile discourses, and associated corporeal practices, can gain greater traction in conditions of persistent social inequality. Being angry or hostile can boost status, ward off threats, and construct tough personae that make attacks and exploitation less likely. Similarly, shame and low status can be reinforced by their associations with and prevalence within the processes of claiming social security benefits, working in devalued occupations, or in social relations generally where inferiority is frequently presumed by others on the basis of accent, clothing, or appearance.

Second, the social and material circumstances of social inequality can themselves induce paranoia, over and above their impact upon relationships. Ross, Mirowsky and Pribesh (2001) found that disadvantaged areas are typically characterised by degrees of disorder, and occupied by relatively powerless communities with low levels of overt mutual trust. People in such areas face an increased risk of assault, theft and burglary, their material environments contain relatively high levels of graffiti, vandalism, and derelict buildings, and street drinking, drug use and visible gangs are all more common. They are also typically subject to greater threat and insecurity because they are more likely to lose their jobs or become homeless, social isolation is often greater, and they have both fewer opportunities and more restricted choices – problems exacerbated by, and causal of, higher levels of ill health. In response to these material threats, people can adopt modes of comportment that decry vulnerability, shame and anxiety and present an appropriately 'hardened' exterior: 'you have to laugh, or else you'll cry' (Millington & Nelson, 1986). And as one of Charlesworth's participants who had recently been made unemployed explained, these threats structure experience:

> I feel different, especially when I go out. Like I'll go for a video or somethin' and when I'm there I feel worried an' threatened a bit, like, an' I sort of can't decide which to have. Then I'll get home and I don't watch it but I'm bored an I need something to do. So I watch it! But I don't enjoy stuff at the moment... nothing seems right to me, not like it was.
>
> (Charlesworth, 1999, p. 77)

Third, relational dynamics, social and material circumstances interact, such that each can amplify the toxic effects of the other. Increased population density, smaller dwellings, greater degrees of social and financial interdependency, and limited resources and opportunities, can mean that the toxic effects of some relationships are felt more keenly. There is extensive evidence that sexual and physical abuse may be causal in psychosis, which frequently includes paranoia: Read et al. (2005) showed that on average 69% of women and 59% of men with psychosis disclose such experiences. There is also research relating male unemployment to physical abuse (Gillham et al., 1998), and showing that the incidence of physical abuse is patterned according to socio-economic and demographic variables (Jack, 2004). Whilst there is no corresponding evidence for sexual abuse, the toxic consequences of both kinds of abuse are likely to be magnified by social inequality, since closer proximity, more shared living space and fewer opportunities for respite or escape mean that contact with the abuser is likely to be more sustained, frequent, prolonged or intense: factors known to make abuse more damaging. Not everyone who is abused experiences clinical paranoia, but abuse nevertheless exemplifies interpersonal situations within which people believe they are not allowed to have or express certain feelings; where having or being seen to have some feelings is dangerous; where it is adaptive not to feel, or at least appear not to feel; or where feelings are difficult to acknowledge because they run counter to the strictures of powerful others. This largely hidden relational variability, and the potentials for shame and disavowal it suggests, reiterates how the contingent associations between social and material conditions and relational dynamics are synergistic, not additive. Not everyone exposed to social inequality experiences clinical paranoia, and nor does everyone who is abused: this kind of interacting variation helps explain why.

## Conclusion

Some of the implications for research and intervention of this kind of analysis have been discussed elsewhere (Cromby & Harper, 2009, 2013). With respect to feelings, the focus on madness exemplifies both their primordially co-constitutive force and the ways in which they can carry the consequences of prior experience across different situations. At the same time, madness highlights again the relations between feeling and rationality, since it is structured by its own acquired logics of feeling that are guided more by social, material and relational circumstance than by conventional reasoning.

# 9
# Concluding

The preceding three chapters showed how an emphasis upon feeling begins to change the way psychology approaches some aspects of a small set of phenomena associated with health and illness. The aim was to demonstrate how the explicit inclusion of feeling extends understanding by uncovering layers of complexity otherwise difficult to discern. With respect to health beliefs, a focus on feeling helps explain not only how belief persists across interactional contexts but also how it gets enacted variably, on a continuum between the extremes of rational reflection and impassioned interjection. With respect to CFS, a focus on feeling helps explain some aspects of this condition and of some ways in which doctor–patient interactions may go awry. Feelings invested on both sides of the medical encounter may, for entirely understandable reasons, get organised as contrasting sensibilities that largely preclude each other's imperatives. And with respect to madness, a focus on feeling illuminates the continuities between the social, the material, the relational and the embodied in lived experiences of distress, helping to explain why madness is consistently associated more with certain combinations of social, relational and material circumstances than with others.

Each of these chapters also introduced concepts that are more generally relevant. Whilst Chapter 6 focused specifically upon health beliefs and the ways in which they might be inculcated and derived, belief figures in many other psychological models and explanations. The concept of believing as an organisation of socialised feeling in contingent articulation with discursive practices and positions therefore has ramifications for many other psychological topics. Similarly, as Chapter 7 acknowledged, the proposition that particular emergent modal sensibilities might be associated with CFS implies that similar or related sensibilities might emerge in relation to other conditions. And, considered more broadly, the concept of a sensibility as an acquired, embodied, pre-reflective orientation may have other implications. For example ideologies – understood as personally lived actualities, rather than formalised abstractions – might be conceived largely as sensibilities. Likewise, the concept of feeling traps, persistent organisations of social, relational and material influence that interpellate complex mixtures of two or more feelings, has many explanatory potentials.

It is appropriate, therefore, to conclude this book by beginning to consider how some of these wider implications might be realised. With this aim in mind, this chapter will first locate the concept of feeling developed here with respect to the broader affective turn with which it is associated. Second, it will situate the psychology of feeling proposed in this book with respect to the broader sphere of psychological knowledge, research and practice.

## The affective turn

Within the affective turn, affect is conceptualised in different ways and is frequently distinguished, at least in part, from both emotion and feeling. Whilst the heterogeneity of this work is such that any generalisation will be to some extent problematic, it seems fair to say that what frequently differentiates affect scholarship from work on emotion is its focus on intensities, forces and flows that exceed and precede the individual. Analyses of affect emphasise communicative, relational and material capacities that forge and shape experience and subjectivity, and are therefore described as autonomous or independent of individual subjects (and indeed, to the extent that affect also animates other organisms, of humans per se). Within this work, concepts of affect get marshalled to index aspects of phenomena that are non-conscious, non- or a-representational, ineffable and virtual, aspects often known only partially through their associated atmospheres or moods. Particularly in work influenced by Deleuze, and hence Spinoza (notably, Massumi's writing), affect is also frequently characterised as vital and undetermined, the essential force and energy of life itself, a raw potentiality known only reductively – once it has been captured and tamed by the sociolinguistic – in its manifestation as emotion and feeling.

The majority of this work, currently, is published beyond the ambit of psychology. Consequently, the most expedient way of relating this research to the concept of feeling developed here will be to consider some of the critiques of the affective turn that were touched upon in the opening chapter. Like any prominent academic movement, the affective turn has attracted various critiques: here, I will briefly summarise the concerns identified by three that seem particularly relevant.

An influential critique by Hemmings (2005) observed that affect scholars sometimes position their work in opposition to poststructuralist and deconstructionist theories of language and its effects. This enables them to highlight how analyses of the discursive structuring of subjectivity effectively dematerialise the body, and so to propose affect as the missing analytic element that brings back the corporeal and material elements of experience. In this way, Hemmings argues, affect is worked up as 'the new cutting edge' that mounts a long-needed challenge to linguistic determinism. Additionally, Hemmings is critical of the way that affect theorists (specifically, in her paper, Sedgwick and Massumi) position affect as an ontological force operating before the sociolinguistic, arguing that this negates epistemological concerns with truth, justice and equality.

Wetherell (2012) is also concerned with the postulated gap or distance between affect and social relations, and in particular with the way that affect frequently gets positioned as before or outside of language. She welcomes and explicitly elaborates upon ways that analyses of affect, emotion or feeling might enrich and be taken up within psychology and social science, supplying lengthy discussions and careful, considered evaluations of the conceptual and evidential resources deployed within this work. Nevertheless, she consistently rejects any suggestion that affect can be theorised or studied independently of its sociolinguistic and discursive mediation, "as an unspecific force, unmediated by consciousness, discourse, representation and interpretation of any kind" (Wetherell, 2012, p. 123). Hence, in place of any sharp disjunction between affect and the sociolinguistic, Wetherell proposes the analysis of contextually situated and para-discursive affective practices.

Perhaps the most damning evaluation of the affective turn is that presented by Leys (2011). Her critique consists of three interrelated strands, the first of which involves challenging the way that basic emotion theories are frequently taken up uncritically within this work. Leys argues that, in relying upon these theories, affect scholars in social science unwittingly reproduce naturalising and reductive assumptions made within psychology and neuroscience. More controversially, perhaps, Leys further argues that in conceptualising affect as 'unqualified intensity' and distinguishing it relatively sharply from emotion, Massumi, Thrift and others generate analyses that are, conceptually and functionally, wholly compatible with the basic emotion paradigm. She draws an equivalence between Deleuzean concepts of affect and psychological concepts of basic emotion, in that what they both share is the presumption of a fundamental disconnection between the powers of affect and the realm of awareness, experience and conventionalised meaning.

Second, Leys argues that this produces a dualism where the body is separated from, and then given precedence, over mind and social relations. An example of this, she argues, is Massumi's discussion of Libet's neuroscientific work on the 'missing half second',[1] which Massumi uses to highlight the significance of corporeal processes outwith and before conscious choice. Whilst Massumi and others use this kind of evidence in a Spinozian/Deleuzian fashion to grant affective powers to the body, Leys argues that by placing affect *before* experience they nevertheless dualistically separate these powers from the cognitive meaning of objects and events.

Third, Leys then argues that these two difficulties together create problems of intentionality or 'aboutness'. Affect is conceptualised as intensity or force before and outside of meaning, and power therefore works ontologically and materially as intensities that – because they precede the sociolinguistic – are necessarily in themselves devoid of meaning, and not intrinsically about anything. Hence, Leys argues, despite the overt political thrust of much of this work, in practice it enacts a paradoxical disconnect between ideology and affect that

> produces as one of its consequences a relative indifference to the role of ideas and beliefs in politics, culture, and art in favour of an 'ontological' concern with different people's corporeal affective reactions.
>
> (Leys, 2011, p. 451)

Whilst these critiques are both telling and grounded in close readings of the texts to which they refer, I want to argue that there is nevertheless still value and utility in affect scholarship; to demonstrate this, two aspects of this work will now be considered in more detail. First, affect theorists usefully emphasise the deliberate or incidental manipulation of material intensities, vibrations or frequencies (which are, most proximally, at their point of impact upon the living body, physiologically transduced). Massumi and others posit that whilst these intensities arise outside of experience they provide some of its constitutive preconditions, and in this way their theorising begins to provide an ontology for the sociocultural. Whilst there is a clear sense in which this ontological thrust is precisely Hemmings' objection, there are also positive aspects to this move. Affect as corporeally sensed intensity highlights a material dimension of experience often downplayed in recent theorising, in psychology as well as in social science; it draws attention to some under-recognised aspects of political dynamics and their processes of influence and control; and it provides a (tentative, partial) bridge between the cultural and the physiological.

Second, affect theorists usefully emphasise the ways that feelings can instantiate in the present the influence of the indeterminate future. For example, Massumi (2010) shows how tension and anxiety can be inculcated and maintained within a political ontology of threat where what could occur in a virtual future becomes an influence in the actual present. By suffusing the present with affective tones of dread reflective of negative or harmful future possibilities, these feelings actualise them as powerful elements of current decision-making. Ideas, images and talk of terror work to constitute an immanent vibratory fabric of tensions and future potentials that impels and structures present political discourse, and which also, and perhaps more significantly, helps secure assent to political practices and surveillance technologies purportedly implemented to neutralise these threats. Importantly, though, virtual futures and their associated feelings are not compelled to be entirely negative and anxiety-laden: as Ellis and Tucker (2011) observe, they can also include hope, the felt index of a positive future yet to be made.

Whilst this book has often concentrated upon feeling as a constituent of experience, it has also argued that bodily potentials need not be consciously experienced to be influential. A relatively straightforward example of this is the disinhibition induced by alcohol consumption, which need not be felt in order to shape activity and experience. A more complex example involves phenomenological habituation to emotional feelings, say in relation to bereavement, where feeling numb and unable to concentrate can take experiential precedence over relationally interpellated mixtures of sadness, anger, fatigue, anxiety and pain. And, more generally, the immediate, a-representational, constitutive character of feeling, its organisation by habit and its frequent interpellation by influences beyond awareness, together lead to a view of consciousness as layered and necessarily lacking complete insight.

We might therefore ask whether it is necessary to institute sharp or permanent distinctions between what is felt and (potentially) sociolinguistically recognised, and what operates beyond experience as affect that necessarily exceeds awareness. Perhaps we can conduct analyses with reference to a notion of feeling which is never reducible to the sociolinguistic but nevertheless runs alongside and within it. If feeling constitutes experience, rather than merely being one of its facets, even unfelt feelings – what Whitehead called negative prehensions – also structure experience, in large part by regulating its material (i.e. biological) substrates. And since the feeling body is always in the world, unfeeling (and its consequences) never happen in a social or relational vacuum. Moreover, the distinctions between what is felt and what is not are frequently dynamic and responsive: what is unfelt at this moment might be felt (again) in the next, only then to – partially, temporarily – recede, oscillations that regulate how feeling influences experience according to how it is organised, impelled, motivated, oriented, directed and interpreted. To illustrate, two examples will now be considered – the first primarily concerned with intensity, the second with future threat.

## Intensifying

Affect scholars frequently consider how affective intensities of various kinds can be inculcated or manipulated in the service of particular goals. For example, Goodman (2012) describes how auditory or sonic intensities are used in military contexts, specifically as weapons, but also as instruments of crowd control. Relatedly, Anderson (2010) discusses how morale in wartime can be manipulated within a 'logistics of affect' wherein, historically at least, voices were prized over text precisely because of their affective connotations. There are conceptual, practical and ideological continuities between these uses of sonic intensity and its deployment within what is politely called forcible (or harsh, or enhanced) interrogation, but more accurately described as torture (Borger, 2014). Military personnel, (from or trained in America, the UK and elsewhere) now routinely use music within interrogation regimes known by chilling euphemisms such as 'fear up harsh', 'futility' and 'pride/ego down'. Most often the music deployed is metal or rap, although other genres and sounds also figure. Typically, the music is played extremely loudly, with the person held in a closely confined space. It may be sustained for periods of days and nights without a break or, alternately, introduced randomly in unexpected deafening bursts (Cusick, 2008). There are at least two sets of sonic intensities at play here: the amplitude or volume, which is so loud that soldiers outside the interrogation cells must shout to each other to be heard; and, where heavy metal is deployed, the clipped high frequency harmonics that sometimes give this music an aggressive and physically painful quality (Pieslak, 2007).

The meanings of these intensities derive initially from their raw qualities of amplitude, harmonics and frequency, temporally manipulated to be either continuous or random. To some extent, intensities thus deployed can work affectively and viscerally at a material or physical level, such that they "ontologically precede the designation of a sensation to a specific exteroceptive sensory channel (the five senses)" (Goodman, 2012, p. 47). They remake experience by systematically innervating the physiology that supports it, so compromising and shaping individual capacities for interpretation and sense making. Powerful, pulsing vibrations of air make chest cavities resonate and visceral organs tremble, invasively imbuing the core of target bodies with rhythmic shivers of raw power whose wholly inescapable medium is the very environment within which the captive is held. Military personnel explicitly recognise these intensive effects, with US Army Psyops spokesperson Ben Abel noting that "It's not so much the music as the sound. It's like throwing a smoke bomb. The aim is to disorient and confuse" (Cusick, 2006, p. 3).[2] Similarly, a British detainee in Guantanamo Bay, Moazzam Begg, has said of his experiences:

> If even footsteps echoed in the building, you can imagine what full blast Marilyn Manson would sound like. Sometimes it would stop at 3 am or so, but your ability to sleep was already disturbed. You lose the ability to have a routine sleep...The other thing that they did was play the music at various times...the random aspect of when it would start or end was frustrating, makes you tired, agitated, upset, on top of all the other situations of not knowing when you're going to be released, interrogated, or moved to those cells. Many people suffered from various kinds of anxiety attacks. People hyperventilated, losing control of their senses, hitting their bottle of water against the cell, against other people, trying to scrape their hands against the concertina wire, sometimes breaking down and crying.
>
> (Cusick, 2008, p. 7)

Whilst the primary focus here is the sonic intensities impelled by music, it is vital to recognise that in forcible interrogation these are routinely supplemented by other intensities, impelled by physical influences directly manipulated by interrogators deploying a variety of techniques. In addition to sonic intensities there are beatings, manipulations of space (confinement), movement (manacles), vision (hooding, goggles, strobe lighting), posture ('stress positions'), respiration ('waterboarding', belts, gags), hearing (ear plugs, white noise), sleep, diet and temperature.

Alongside the effects of its sonic intensities, music in interrogation also bears more conventionalised meanings that may further enhance its force. Cusick (2006) observes that, to those largely unversed in their nuances and codes, rap and metal music can readily be heard as embodying the sound of masculine rage. Arabic music, which can be particularly offensive to devout Muslims, is sometimes used (Pieslak, 2007); as is music featuring sexually expressive female vocalists (notably, Cristina Aguilera) which seems calculated to offend religious sensibilities (Cusick, 2008). More plaintively, few can be surprised that when subjected to a continuous loud recording of babies crying "detainees usually answered questions after a half hour of listening" (Pieslak, 2007, p. 132). But interrogators also interspersed these choices with brief interludes of calming and possibly familiar or reassuring music, with the apparent goal of inducing crippling self-pity: "they played an artist I enjoyed. But that just... began destroying me. Listening to songs that I would play at home... within that place, drove me to tears" (Cusick, 2008, p. 22).

Some other possible layers of meaning are prefigured cinematically. Roy Orbison sings about the candy-coloured clown they call the sandman whilst a man is savagely beaten; a gangster sings along to 'Stuck in the Middle With You' whilst slicing off a man's ear. Music during interrogation might similarly signal that, for the interrogator, this is a relaxed activity with distinct capacities for play and enjoyment: a troubling signal likely to magnify dread and erode hope. At the same time, making music into a weapon involves transforming a familiar element of domestic life into something utterly sinister, a transformation that begins to fundamentally unravel civilised existence.[3] And, taking a still broader perspective, Cusick (2008) observes that the material nature of amplified music as acoustic energy, derived from electrical energy and archetypally produced at 'black sites' by oil-fired generators, functions in contemporary wars – where oil is frequently implicated – to reinforce dominance through the spectacular use of the very resource most obviously at stake.

In forcible interrogation, then, sonic intensities are typically paralleled by other intensities apprehended through multiple perceptual channels. These intensities produce visceral, felt embodied signs already imbued with a primordial intentionality reflective of their somatic character: pain, trembling, insomnia, fatigue, hunger, breathlessness, sensory deprivation and sensory overload. These primordial meanings then get enrolled with others: those suggested by the meanings of the music played, and by the mere playing of music in such contexts. What is more, *all* of these various signs and meanings are to a great extent *already* intentional by virtue of their occurrence within profoundly intimidating material-relational situations starkly suggestive of future threat, such as

> a 'dark prison' filled with deafening Western music. The lights were barely turned on...One man shouted at him through an interpreter, 'You are in a place that is out of the world. No-one knows where you are, no-one is going to defend you'.
>
> (Cusick, 2008, p. 1)

As Scarry (1985) observes, torture differs from everyday experiences of pain in terms of its duration (typically more extensive), its relationship to control (the captive typically has none), and its purpose (which is wholly malign). The intensive meanings of the discomfort, anxiety and disorientation produced by painfully loud and unpleasant music are therefore already modulated by the captive's pre-existing relationship to the interrogators, a relationship enacted within a significantly larger interplay of punishment, control and domination that ultimately instantiates grand fictions of domination.[4] Consequently, in forcible interrogation sonic intensities supply but one aspect of an entire complex of meanings, the combined effects of which – as Guantanamo detainee Mohamedou Ould Slahi explains – can induce states of madness such as those described in the previous chapter:

> I started to hallucinate and hear voices as clear as crystal. I heard my family in a casual family conversation...I heard Qur'an readings in a heavenly voice. I heard music from my country. Later on the guards used these hallucinations and started talking with funny voices through the plumbing, encouraging me to hurt the guard and plot an escape.
>
> (Ackerman & Cobain, 2015)

Notwithstanding the levels of detail here, it must be emphasised that what can be known of the effects of music during interrogation is partial. Before release, detainees are typically compelled to sign confidentiality agreements, any breach of which renders them liable to immediate re-arrest and confinement: understandably, few speak openly of their experiences. It nevertheless seems clear that, to the extent that the effects of the sonic intensities marshalled by interrogators can be understood alone, they serve to impel feelings of confusion, fatigue, misery, weakness and anxiety. However, it is also clear that these sonic intensities do not function in isolation. Rather, they are continuously enrolled and amplified within simultaneous overlapping layers of meaning jointly worked up somatically, materially, psychologically and socially. This is not to say that, ontologically, there is no purely affective-sonic level upon which intensity operates: simply to acknowledge that its effects are always simultaneously refracted through both a human body and a humanly constituted sphere of power relations, practice and sociolinguistic meaning. Additionally, rather than the sociolinguistic working to tame and capture the intensive, as Massumi suggests, in forcible interrogation it frequently works additively or synergistically to magnify its force.

## Threatening

The affective politics and corporeal practices of forcible interrogation may seem quite remote to the great majority of the populace, who do not imagine that such a fate could ever befall them. The everyday machinations of governance and politics consist largely of mundane performance (the TV interview, the parliamentary speech, the party political broadcast, the manifesto) designed to inculcate felt sensibilities manifesting acquiescence or compliance, such that for much of the time we are simultaneously both subject to banal power and make of ourselves banal subjects of power (c.f. Hook, 2007) Certainly, there is no moral equivalence between the everyday actions of contemporary politicians seeking to gain or maintain power and the actions of torturers.[5] At the same time, however, the putative threats to which interrogators respond – threats of terror, of terrorism, of war, violence and subversion – are prominent amongst the many threats that contemporary politicians identify, mobilise and exploit in their everyday political practice.

In recent years a series of analysts have argued that political power and authority is increasingly legitimated on the basis of threats, fears and anxieties. Glassner (1999) and Baumann (2006) both accord fear a central role in the emotional dynamics of contemporary Anglo-American cultures. Stearns (2008) suggests that in America since the 1930's a new emotional standard has gradually emerged so that instead of confronting and challenging fear, politicians now incite it for their own ends. He proposes that this is possible primarily because of three factors: the 'crisis saturation' of recent history, the impact of the news media, and altered patterns of child socialisation. A study by Franklin (2011) concluded that parenting and childcare in the UK are also frequently infused by and oriented towards fear and threat. Similarly, Furedi (2007) argues that contemporary governmentality operates within an affective dynamic he calls a culture of fear. This culture is characterised by features including risk aversion, a 'new etiquette' where logics of good and bad have been largely supplanted by considerations of safety and danger. Risk, both actual and hypothetical, is omnipresent, producing a continuous orientation towards 'health and safety'. This culture is materially rooted in a series of changes that include transformations of production and employment and associated patterns of living that have shattered formerly stable bonds of community, the rise of 'no win, no fee' legal practices, and the growth of a rolling 24-hour news media always hungry for another headline.

The incitement of threat in the service of governmentality has non-incidental material concomitants. In recent decades the UK government has equipped itself with a technological infrastructure of surveillance and control (CCTV, automatic number plate and face recognition cameras, biometric passports, bulk interception of phone calls, emails and internet activity) sufficient to enable a future totalitarian state. Moreover, as the disclosures of security services whistle-blower Edward Snowden show (Greenwald, 2014), the UK is not alone in implementing such technologies. This infrastructure inculcates its own 'affective atmosphere', positioning individuals in a felt tension between discourses of privacy and security such that surveillance can be experienced ambivalently, as both threatening and reassuring (Ellis, Tucker, & Harper, 2013). Threat and fear also impel the political trajectories that depend upon them, such that they become mutually sustaining. Within days of the January 2015 murder in Paris of 12 journalists at the satirical magazine 'Charlie Hebdo' (with its ensuing manhunt and further associated casualties), UK Prime Minister David Cameron (echoing the head of MI5, Andrew Parker) called for additional new powers to be granted to the security services – even though evidence suggests that such powers would not have prevented either the French attack or recent UK atrocities including the murder of Lee Rigby and the 2005 London bombings (Norton-Taylor, 2015).

It should nevertheless be noted that fear is not the only feeling incited and organised within contemporary governance. There is a sense in which, to a significant extent, the workings of ideology involve the interpellation, manipulation, suppression, organisation, chaining and finessing of feeling more generally. Ideology – in the guise of rhetoric, its most frequent practical manifestation – frequently implicates practices of association, repetition and direction between feeling and signification. Certain feelings get repeatedly associated with these objects rather than those: anger with 'benefit scroungers' rather than bankers (Cromby & Willis, 2014), admiration with venture capitalist 'dragons' rather than campaigners for equality, and resentment with immigrants taking low paid jobs rather than employers paying low wages. These associations get repeated, in different registers, media and terminologies, over and again: sometimes as arguments or incitements, sometimes as facts attributed to experts and sometimes nuanced by other felt associations that neutralise or blur their otherwise totalising tendencies, so rendering the overall pattern less perceptible. We are thus incited not only to feel but to unfeel – to feel empathy, for example, only selectively, and in relation to specific approved others (Olson, 2012). Feeling gets publicly channelled and directed primarily in accord with dominant interests, and – because feeling constitutes and impels experience – attention, contemplation, analysis and action frequently follow.

The culture of fear infuses politics, not just as routine governmentality, but also as ideology. On 11th February 2003, the Blair government in the UK deployed tanks outside London Heathrow Airport, in response to what they claimed was a very specific and 'chilling' terrorist threat. The government, who claimed to have intelligence that a terrorist attack on London was not only probable but 'imminent' (Bamber, Craig, & Elliott, 2003), ensured that this dramatic military action gained substantial media coverage: nevertheless, no attack materialised. Whilst the anti-Iraq War demonstration that took place in London a few days later on 15 February 2003 was the largest protest in UK history, it is only possible to speculate how much bigger it might have been were it not for not this spectacular intervention.

Relatedly, Massumi (2010) analyses how the second Bush government in the USA frequently legitimated its military actions in Iraq by inciting fear. Ranging across examples such as Saddam Hussein's elusive weapons of mass destruction, an airport incident where white flour was mistaken for anthrax poison, and the whole of New York city being placed on terror alert in October 2005 due to a 'chillingly specific' threat to bomb its transport systems (a threat never realised), Massumi demonstrates that allusions and incitements of fear frequently become more real than the putative objects or events to which they refer. His analyses show how:

> The felt reality of the threat is so superlatively real that it translates into a felt certainty about the world, even in the absence of other

grounding for it in the observable world. The assertion has the felt
certainty of a 'gut feeling'.

(Massumi, 2010, p. 55)

These examples demonstrate that the claim from affect theory that contemporary politicians incite and manage collective fears and anxieties
by enrolling past and future threats within discourses and practices of
governance is well founded. In this, the insight that virtual futures can
get actualised in the present as feelings of tension and anxiety offers
a novel insight into the dynamics of power. Nevertheless, even more so
than with the example of forcible interrogation, it seems clear that none
of this requires a notion of affect as a non-intentional force or capacity wholly outwith the sociolinguistic. In the invocation of threatening
futures, the divides between what is felt, what is represented and talked
about, and what is either unfelt or known only as a kind of vague corporeal intensity (such as a gut feeling), are continuously crossed. Indeed, it
is notable that – at least this analysis – Massumi himself returns affect
to feeling. Not only does he talk explicitly of feelings (as in the quote
above) he also relates their operation – and in particular their seeming
ability to be influential without entering awareness – to Whitehead's
notion of negative prehensions (i.e. of what is eliminated from feeling
in the production of experience).

At this point the arguments begin to come full circle. Bodily intensities not reducible to the sociolinguistic can indeed contribute to
meaning (and this is something with which Langer would surely have
agreed). Yet even where these intensities are directly and explicitly
manipulated under the highly controlled conditions of interrogation,
they do not operate independently of signification and social practice.
Whilst intensities have a force of their own, their force is always exerted
in and known through the realm of lived human experience. Moreover,
in becoming influential intensities are typically at least partially felt:
albeit that this partiality is engendered at least as much by entrained
physiologies (which, for example, subtract the audibly acoustic from
the material realm of sonic vibration) as by processes of capture within
normative sociolinguistic grids.

Similarly, virtual futures instantiated as present actualities are known
corporeally as feelings, but both their interpellation, and the ways in
which their significances are stabilised, flow through and work with the
sociolinguistic, rather than simply bypassing or undercutting it. The
sociolinguistic works not so much to capture or tame affect or feeling as to incite, articulate and mobilise it, in the service of interests

that arrange its conjunctions in ways reflective of dominant ideological forces.

To summarise: the focus on intensities beyond and constitutive of practices of signification and modes of experience does reveal some aspects of the operation of power and the influence of materiality. However, the effects of these intensities are only ever known within wider spheres of meaning and significance, even if they are not wholly reducible to them. Moreover, the influence of the virtual, the ways in which it is made to matter as precisely this feeling rather than that (e.g. as dread rather than hope) actually *requires* the sociolinguistic, not just as medium of analysis but also as a vital vehicle for its operation. On this basis, the postulated gap between affect and meaning seems unnecessary: analyses might equally be based upon a notion of feeling as it primordially constitutes experience in ways that precede, but are not separate from, our more conventionalised ways of knowing.

## Psychology

In order to situate psychological analyses of feeling with respect to the wider discipline of psychology, three overlapping issues likely to be encountered by a psychology of feeling will be considered: humanism, individualism and interiority. The dangers these issues might provoke are described, and ways in which they might be neutralised are suggested.

The first issue is humanism, which is a perspective rather than a coherent philosophy or movement (Burston, 2014). In psychology, humanism is associated with a tendency to prioritise the human within both ethics and ontology[6] and to thus treat experience as transparently available for interrogation, rational reflection and self-report. With respect to feeling, humanism lurks within analyses that identify emotions or feelings as analytic objects but without endorsing any theorisation of them, therefore reproducing humanist assumptions about their character.

In this context, a clear strength of the account presented here is that it is specifically *human* without being *humanist*. Feeling is provided for us by our bodies. It is not simply within our control, and nor – because it is ineffable, a-representational, fundamentally not a matter of formal symbolism – is it even necessarily capable of being rendered wholly sensible in ways that we can communicate to others. This is also in part because any sense we do make will necessarily be influenced by the feelings concurrent with the interpretation, which may not be

identical with the prior feeling we are striving to interpret: this generates a perpetual circularity and layers of complexity which confound
privileged insight. It is also because, in our activity of making sense
of feeling, we must 'cut into' its ineffable flow, we necessarily have to
artificially 'fix' upon one relatively bounded aspect of its duration to
turn it into something stable enough to be represented and reflected
upon. But this fixing or stabilisation is transformative, in two ways.
First, because it necessarily involves freezing something that is always
moving; second, because it renders into the realm of discourse or symbol a primordial element of experience that is fundamentally neither
discursive nor symbolic.

Add to this Langer's observation that the majority of feeling states
pass fleetingly, transiently, without ever being represented or conceptualised and it seems very clear that feeling need not implicate a rational,
self-aware subject possessing accurate and comprehensive insight. The
humanist ideology that explains social life on the basis of the conscious
intentions and plans of bounded, rational, controlling social actors, is
incompatible with a fluid, process account which has a-representational
feelings at its core. Simultaneously, Langer's account is specifically
*human* in that a central thrust of her work is to establish and account
for what she calls the 'great shift' from animal to human mentality, a
qualitative shift from what she sees as the instinctive acts of animals to
the conceptually registered acts of humans.[7]

The second issue is individualism: the psychological tendency to
first imagine that we can meaningfully separate individuals from the
collectives that co-constitute their experience, and then to prioritise
these already-mythical individuals within analyses and explanations.
It was suggested in Chapter 1 that psychology is in part structured,
and therefore dominated, by deep tendencies towards different kinds of
individualism, including (as Chapter 5 argued) the enduring methodological individualism associated with quantitative and experimental
research. Consequently, individualism is a pervasive problem for psychology in general, which frequently positions individuals as the singular source and origin of their experiences and actions. And feeling,
of course, is experienced individually. However much it might be both
socialised and relationally and situationally interpellated, its movements and significances are known in their fullness only within the
intimacy of embodied experience. In the context of a discipline deeply
predicated upon individuals understood as essentially separate from others, this means that a psychology of feeling will inevitably encounter
pulls towards individualism.

These pulls can be resisted if it is recognised, first, that feeling is provided for us by our bodies whether we wish it or not: it is not a matter of individual will or choice. Second, many feelings are interpellated by the situations we move through, situations whose meanings are co-constituted for each of us, not just by their present characteristics, but also by the entrained memories and habitually felt associations they simultaneously impel. And third, as the evidence and discussions in Chapter 3 demonstrated, feelings of all kinds get pre-reflectively socialised within regimes of practice associated with specific cultural norms. These regimes produce somatic repertoires associated with sociological variables such as SES and gender and simultaneously inflected and mediated by more variable and proximal influences transmitted in parenting, family and employment. This is why Chapter 4 argued that individuality is best understood as radical individuality – in its absolute cultural-historical-biological uniqueness, but more tellingly in that it is constituted from elements, resources and tendencies entirely shared with others, and only temporarily ring-fenced within the individual subjectivities they constitute.

The third issue likely to be encountered by a psychology of feeling is interiority: the tendency to consider the internal dynamics of experience and subjectivity separately from the situations and circumstances within which they occur. Whilst there is a sense in which interiority is largely what psychology analyses it is also an issue more generally. With relation to affect scholarship, for example, Clough (2010) suggests that, because of their emphasis upon autopoiesis, even analyses predicted upon relational ontologies tend to at least implicitly reproduce relatively fixed boundaries between self and other, and hence to imply relatively bounded interior dynamics within each. Consequently, interiority highlights the danger that a psychology of feeling might tend to unwittingly reproduce mainstream psychological preoccupations with processes, attributes and characteristics presumed to reside and operate wholly inside individuals, who then get understood as pristine solitary centres of mental activity.

In the face of this danger, it is necessary to recall that feeling – as process, rather than entity – is pre-reflectively socialised and continuously relational and responsive. Whilst Langer categorised feeling as either autogenous or exogenous, as emotion or as sensation, she also worded her distinction with reference to how feeling is *experienced*, rather than with reference to any absolute ontological difference. Additionally, as Innis (2009, p. 226) says, for Langer acts intervene upon acts in unexpected and powerful ways, overriding the pivotal distinction running through Langer's thought of peripheral impact, coming from outside, and autogenic action, originating from within. In one sense our own thoughts can interrupt our 'train of thoughts'. The inside has its own outside, and can feel the supervenient thought as impact.

Thus, in the twin dialectics between feeling and inner speech, on the one hand, and experience and social relations on the other, words both spoken and unspoken – and indeed, memories, fantasies and dreams – may not only 'complete' prior pulses of feeling, but also impel new ones. The intimate dynamics of embodied experience are already enmeshed with the public dynamics of relating, interacting, choosing, deciding, talking, listening and acting. Within these dynamics, the liminality of feeling, its status as an emergent aspect of the living body that co-constitutes experience both in and through social relations, makes it an ideal candidate for analyses that do not pre-emptively separate interior from exterior, individual from social, nature from culture or body from mind.

# Notes

## 1 Introducing

1. Even in Anglo-American cultures, in its everyday experience disgust seems to be not so much wholly distinct and encapsulated as on a continuum or spectrum that also includes experiences which we might call distaste, disdain, revulsion, condescension, scorn and contempt (Highmore, 2010).
2. A definition more typically expressed as 'the capacity to affect and to be affected'. The circularity here is more apparent than real, since it reflects the process character of notions of affect: nevertheless, an alternative wording was used in order to minimise confusion.
3. A further discussion of the affective turn, and the critiques addressing it, appears in Chapter 9.
4. Within the change of metaphor, cognitive psychology inherited from behaviourism the notion of organisms as something like a switchbox with inputs and outputs. In behaviourism, the interest was primarily in stimulus and response per se, whereas in cognitivism the interest was in the flow of information that led from one to the other – as, for example, in the TOTE (test–operate–test–exit) model of cognitive regulation. Thus, within the metaphorical transformation from behaviourism to cognitivism, from mechanical machine to information processing device, there are continuities as well as differences.
5. References within this book to 'our' culture should be consistently read as referring to English-speaking, Anglo-American cultures. I have avoided the more typical designation of 'Western' culture both because of its inaccuracy and imprecision (does it include or exclude the English speaking global south?) and because of the Orientalist contrast upon which it depends. Many thanks to Darrin Hodgetts for his helpful comments on this.
6. "Every discipline has its 'black boxes' on which basic arguments depend, but whose contents we either take for granted or believe, mistakenly, to be in the safe custody of some other discipline" (Robertson 2001, p. 106).
7. "For the living subject his own body might well be different from all external objects: the fact remains that for the unsituated thought of the psychologist the experience of the living subject became itself an object and, far from requiring a fresh definition of being, took its place in universal being" (Merleau-Ponty, 2002, p. 108).

## 2 Feeling

1. Langer challenges the Darwinian account of evolution because, in her view, it gives the organism an overly passive role. She argues that natural selection "is a historical pattern, not a mechanism" (1967 p. 394). The mechanisms or causes of evolution, she proposes, are the acts of an organism

as it advances within a dialectic between individuation (separating and distinctiveness) and involvement (inclusion and interpenetration), a dialectic where both processes occur within a specified niche or environment, an ambient.

2. However, Innis (2009) finds that there are also metaphysical elements within Langer's analysis of mind.

3. "[C]onsciousness is the crown of experience, only occasionally attained, not its necessary base" (Whitehead, 1927, p. 267).

4. Wilson (2004) considers how the gut contains so many serotonin receptors that some neuroscientists call it the 'second brain'. She uses this evidence to challenge the presumption that cognition and understanding are solely enabled by the brain. She argues that recognising the gut's continuous contribution to cognition and judgement illuminates various aspects of everyday experience whilst also producing a more sophisticated and accurate account of cognition itself.

5. Damasio's (1999) concept of consciousness as "the feeling of what happens" has various interesting parallels with Langer's, notwithstanding that he emphasises difference rather than intensity as the productive basis of experience.

6. Superficially, at least, it is paradoxical to identify feelings as an analytical category separate from emotions and partially constituted as a component of them, yet at the same time to talk of feelings of anger, shame, fear and the like. However, this apparent paradox might itself be considered largely the product of a prior naturalistic conception of emotion. We might instead assume some degree of socio-cultural co-constitution: that emotions are always hybrids of the kind that Prinz (2004) posits. From this perspective, talk of feelings of shame, anger, fear or any other emotion recognises, on the one hand, that these experiences have a marked somatic component and on the other hand, that this somaticity is developed and shaped by experience within a particular socio-cultural arena that serves to give it meaning and relevance. Hence to talk of 'feelings of anger' is to deploy shorthand for a complex of socio-somatic processes with currency in our culture. For a sociological analysis of the extent to which emotions are socio-culturally invariant, see Turner (2000).

7. Feelings of pain can themselves be further categorised, for example, along the dimensions embedded within the McGill Pain Questionnaire, to draw out qualities such as their rhythmicity or temporality, and their thermal and constrictive dimensions (Scarry, 1985)

8. There is an echo here of the Zajonc–Lazarus debate over whether prior cognition is necessary for affect. Zajonc supplied evidence suggesting that "preferences need no inferences", showing that mere exposure to an unfamiliar symbol such as a Chinese ideograph increased the subsequent likelihood that this particular ideograph would be chosen from an array and rated more positively. Lazarus disputed Zajonc's interpretation of these experiments and supplied evidence of his own, which suggested that prior cognitive appraisal is a necessary pre-requisite for affect to occur.

9. In scholarship associated with the affective turn, the term 'affect' is often deployed precisely in order to index these pre-reflective, extra-experiential aspects of feeling: see the discussions in Chapters 1 and 9.

# 3 Relating

1. Although Voronov and Singer (2002) question the evidence for this distinction.
2. The term 'epigenetics' has recently changed its dominant meaning. Contemporary epigenetic research is less concerned with heritability and, instead, is focused more on the ways in which gene expression is modulated by environmental influences as they get embedded within biological processes.
3. An academic fashion that, as current neoliberal policies bite deeper, might now be changing somewhat (see e.g. McKenzie, 2015).
4. If class is understood as a relationship within the means of production reflective of degrees of ownership and control, then this fundamental economic relation has not been eradicated. Likewise, if class is understood in terms of the embodiment of social capital, it is clear that whilst the contents and style of this embodiment might have changed in some respects, differences in status and power have intensified in recent years. The apolitical celebration of difference and concomitant promotion of identity and choice seem to reflect the dominance of neoliberalism, notwithstanding that they might also provide the seeds of other ways of being.
5. Similar debates are also arising in social neuroscience, although there is some disagreement about their terms; for example, implicit versus explicit, reflexive versus reflective and 'system 1' versus 'system 2' (see Adolphs, 2010).

# 4 Experiencing

1. "Thought is not expressed but completed in the word" (Vygotsky, 1962, p. 250).
2. At the end of *Thought and Language*, Vygotsky (1962, p. 271) says, "Thought and speech turn out to be the key to the nature of human consciousness."
3. Langer's evolutionary account of mind posits a yet more fundamental dialectic of experience between autogenic and external feeling, between what is experienced as subjective and what is experienced as objective. She proposes that in evolved humans 'every internal feeling tends to issue in a symbol which gives it an objective status, even if only transiently' (Langer, 1972, p. 342). Vygotsky's account of inner speech suggests a specific means, whereby language enters into, contributes to and thus transforms this dialectic.
4. Langer argues that the evolution of thinking was driven in part by 'overstimulation' of the brain that results in the completion of value-laden acts in the form of (mental) images: "the symbolic finishing of excessive nervous impulses within the nervous system itself...begets the first processes of ideation" (Langer, 1972, p. 314). Mental activity is the incredibly complex outcome of multiple concurrent processes of increasing complexity where lower processes get entrained by higher ones, and feeling is never separate from symbolisation. The suggestion here is that what we call emotion occurs as a specific phase in these processes, typically characterised either by excessive intensity or normative disjunction.

5. 'When we converse with ourselves, we need even fewer words... Inner speech is speech almost without words' (Vygotsky, 1962, p. 258)
6. This is an example of a feeling trap – see Chapter 8.
7. It seems possible that some feelings of knowing could also be produced in other ways, for example, simply by temporarily or transiently associating aspects of bodies of socially acquired knowledge with sensori-motor feelings of the kind that Johnson (2007) posits to be important.
8. The recurrence of related kinds of emotion across history and culture need not necessarily imply specific kinds of genetic predetermination in the manner of basic emotion theories. Some degree of commonality might be accounted for on the basis of frequently recurring social and organisational forms (e.g. families, collectives, hierarchies) that generate cross-cultural potentials for quite similar normative breaches and overspills of feeling.
9. And, to this extent, they are probably not identical with the affective practices described by Wetherell (2012). This is because, whilst on my reading she is somewhat inconclusive on this issue, it seems that Wetherell primarily wants to approach these practices largely through analyses of language.
10. "In inner speech... a single word is so saturated with sense that it becomes a concentrate of sense. To unfold it into overt speech, one would need a multitude of words" (Vygotsky, 1962, p. 262).
11. Cognitive psychology sometimes references notions of cognitive effort that superficially index some of the experiential elements Langer identifies, but re-conceptualises them in wholly computational terms as "the engaged proportion of limited-capacity central processing" (Tyler et al., 1979, p. 607). This considerably downplays the extent to which the strains and labour of thinking are already a matter of feeling.
12. 'Subjectivity' is a term with an intellectual lineage descending from sources that include Marxism, poststructuralism, phenomenology and psychoanalysis (Blackman, L., Cromby, J., Hook, D., Papadopoulos, D., & Walkerdine, V., 2008). It indexes the same phenomena that psychology conceptualises as self or personality, but its allegiance to those alternative traditions of thought largely neutralises the individualism and liberal humanism that these notions reproduce.
13. There is here perhaps an issue of academic taste that reflects the material position and liberal leanings of the majority of academics and which – in not recognising and engaging on their own terms those aspects of working-class culture that reject middle-class norms – can even effectively function in ways largely indistinguishable from dismissal of or even contempt for them (see Charlesworth, 1999).

## 5   Researching

1. It must be emphasised that the CAS is neither intrinsically better nor worse than many other questionnaire-based self-report measures of emotion; its use as an example here simply reflects its accessibility and relevance.
2. A highly respected colleague once told me that their usual response to objections to quantitative research, raised within critical psychological and qualitative methodological writings, was simply to think "So why don't you just fuck off and do your own research?"

3. Relatedly, Langer notes the evidence that children pass through a phase of 'physiognomic' perception where "overall qualities of fearfulness, friendliness, serenity etc. seem to characterise objects more naturally than their physical constitution" (Langer, 1967, pp. 132–133). And similarly, Merleau-Ponty (2002, p. 25) says, "When we come back to phenomena we find, as a basic layer of experience, a whole already pregnant with an irreducible meaning: not sensations with gaps between them, into which memories may be supposed to slip, but the features, the layout of a landscape or a word, in spontaneous accord with the intentions of the moment, as with earlier experience."
4. Perhaps another way of stating this problem is that in not theorising emotion, qualitative researchers – at least implicitly – draw upon the same reductive, biologistic notions mobilised by affect theorists (see Leys, 2011; see also Chapter 9 in this volume).

# 6  Believing

1. Cytokines are small proteins involved in the signalling processes between cells that regulate their behaviour; pro-inflammatory cytokines are proteins that promote systemic inflammation.
2. Hence, in the UK some members of the racist political party the National Front saw no apparent contradiction between their being avowed party members and simultaneously having black friends (Billig, 1978).
3. Simplifying hugely, for Whitehead propositions are hybrids composed of 'actual entities' and 'pure potentialities'. Whitehead (1927, p. 256) describes propositions as "the tales that might be told of particular actualities". Hence, in combining what there is with a primitive feel for what might be enabled by what there is, propositions serve to lure feelings in specific directions.
4. This might especially be the case where beliefs are acquired very early in life. Bucci (1997) posits the existence of subsymbolic memories for emotional experiences, memories that can be acquired before, or in the absence of, language or any other symbol system. Such feeling-laden memories might impel powerful, deep-rooted beliefs that their possessors nevertheless struggle to recognise or articulate.

# 7  Exhausting

1. No assumptions of any kind will be made here about the status and causes of CFS, and the analysis does not commit to any particular theory about its ontogenesis.
2. The websites were:

   (1) http://www.supportme.co.uk/
   (2) http://www.nhsdirect.nhs.uk/en.asp?TopicID=121
   (3) http://www.rcpsych.ac.uk/info/mhgu/newmhgu33.htm
   (4) http://www.bbc.co.uk/health/ask_doctor/chronic_fatigue_syndrome.shtml
   (5) http://www.bbc.co.uk/health/conditions/chronicfatigue.shtml
   (6) http://www.kcl.ac.uk/cfs/

(7) http://hcd2.bupa.co.uk/fact_sheets/html/chronic_fatigue_syndrome2
.html

(8) http://www.psychnet-uk.com/dsm_iv/chronic_fatigue_syndrome.htm

(9) http://www.parliament.uk/commons/ lib/research/rp98/rp98–107.pdf

(10) http://www.netdoctor.co.uk/special_reports/depression/cfs.htm

(11) http://www.cfs-news.org/

(12) http://www.cfids-me.org/

(13) http://www.afme.org.uk/

(14) http://www.thesite.org/youthnet/jsp/polopoly.jsp?d=162&a=330

(15) http://web.ukonline.co.uk/ruth.livingstone/little/cfs1.htm

(16) http://www.ivillage.co.uk/health/ghealth/discon/articles/0,,181033
_182772,00.html

(17) http://www.nmec.org.uk/

(18) http://www.rcpsych.ac.uk/publications/cr/cr54.htm

3. CFS is not 'really' masked or anxious depression, but this is not because its medical aspects can be divorced from its subjective, felt or experiential aspects. It is because neither depression nor CFS has any biological pathology consistently associated with them, and in that sense neither is more true or real than the other. At the same time, both diagnoses are real cultural accomplishments that simultaneously reflect and impel extant organisations of experience. Asserting that one 'is' the other means the unwarranted promotion of one or other diagnostic category over these nuances of experience, a reifying move that largely glosses how different concatenations of social, material and relational influence differentially organise the feelings, discourses and practices typically associated with each diagnosis (and indeed with both).

4. The ways in which mixtures of these covert biological and societal influences might combine and intersect to reproduce ideologies and power hierarchies is a topic frequently considered within analyses of affect (see Chapter 9).

# 8  Maddening

1. At no point should this analysis be misread as family blaming. This allegation – often used to discredit critics of psychiatry – rests upon a series of mistaken assumptions and inferences. Families function as complex systems wherein agency cannot simply be attributed to individuals. Family members very rarely intend to drive others mad, do not necessarily know the consequences of their actions and are frequently doing the best they can to manage distress or toxic circumstances of their own. Whilst families frequently loom massively in the experience of their members, children especially, their degrees of actual power in the wider world are typically very limited. Families therefore function largely as conduits for wider distal forces and influences, constantly shaped and buffeted by greater powers for which – in relation to their constituent members – they are merely the medium. The descrying of relational explanations for madness as mere family blaming is therefore not only overly simplistic, it also substitutes a moral-pragmatic argument for a scientific one (for which there is extensive evidence), disingenuously seeking to align family members with psychiatry in the process.

2. Whilst Scheff largely naturalises shame in his analyses, other scholars deconstruct some of its meanings. Leys (2007) contrasts what she describes as the anti-mimetic tendencies of shame with the identificatory or mimetic qualities of guilt. Agamben (2002) draws upon Levinas to relate shame to intimacy and the inability to lose focus upon oneself. These analysts nevertheless largely agree with Scheff's view of the great and under-recognised significance of shame in everyday life.

3. The 2004 film *Downfall* brilliantly portrays these two alternating aspects of Hitler's character.

4. Healy (1987) proposed that dysentrainment produced by disrupted relationships and material circumstances – losing a job, ending a relationship, being bereaved – might produce many of the experiences associated with the diagnosis of depression.

5. Freeman et al.'s work comes superficially close to overcoming this problem by positing that delusions are the direct consequence of emotional states, such that anxiety "contains a cognitive component 'anticipation of danger'" (2006, p. 563) and that "cognitive-affective biases" or "emotion-related cognitive biases" (2013, p. 1281) are the root cause of paranoid delusions: nevertheless, even here there is still a dichotomy between thought and emotion, rather than a differentiated continuum. Bentall's model, by contrast, appears more thoroughly cognitive, with the interplay between attributions and self-representations being the main driver of delusional thinking.

6. Whilst Trower and Chadwick's model seems less problematic because it adopts a biographical process stance toward paranoid delusions, implicit tendencies toward stasis still arise because of the way it largely separates emotion from cognition and it's manifestations, including belief.

7. Feinstein et al. (2002, p. 1258) speculate that their study "is consistent with the hypothesis that the prefrontal cortex filters out emotionally irrelevant information by inhibiting the amygdala".

8. "[Anxiety] is an existential predicament, absorption ceases, and life seems like a game with no meaning. A life without public embedding in which these people must put forward an endless pretence, to the Department of Social Security, to potential employers, their lives are criss-crossed with regimes, regimes aimed at disavowing the truth their experience asserts in the face of a veil of public lies. Little wonder the matterings of life become problematic, and little wonder many feel sick and unsettled. The everyday practical lives of their communities have become fractured, and with them the sources of respect and value available have fallen away, leaving this amorphous sense of discomfort, unease and anxiety" (Charlesworth, 1999, p. 80).

## 9  Concluding

1. Libet presented a series of experiments within which people were asked to report the moment they decided to respond to a stimulus by pressing a lever. His measures of brain activity seemed to show that preparatory surges of sensori-motor activity preceded the conscious decision to act by around 400 milliseconds. Whilst the finding is relatively robust its interpretation – by

Libet, and by others including Massumi – is less clear and, as Leys demonstrates, need not be taken to mean that action is simply decided by the body before it is chosen by the mind.

2. In this instance, Abel was speaking specifically about the use of music within battlefield deployments; nevertheless, the more general point still holds.

3. "Made to participate in the annihilation of the prisoners, made to demonstrate that everything is a weapon, the objects themselves, and with them the fact of civilisation, are annihilated" (Scarry, 1985, p. 41).

4. "[P]hysical pain is so incontestably real that it seems to confer its quality of 'incontestable reality' on that power that has brought it into being. It is, of course, precisely because the reality of that power is so highly contestable, the regime so unstable, that torture is being used" (Scarry, 1985, p. 27).

5. Albeit that the torturers are often working on behalf of those same politicians to implement practices of discipline and punishment portrayed largely as information-gathering.

6. And, more broadly, with uses of the category 'human' to warrant colonial exploitation.

7. For Langer, this shift is impelled by many forces, key amongst which is an accumulation and differentiation of movements of feeling, enabled by increasingly capable neural systems. Once these movements begin to realise their potential as mental images rather than physical actions, what we call imagination begins and symbolisation, most obviously through language but also in art, then follows. However, other elements also contribute, including both the capacity to remember and the possibility of using language to order memory.

# References

Ackerman, S., & Cobain, I. (2015, 17 January). From inside Guantanamo, a tale of torture and torment. *The Guardian*.

Adolphs, R. (2010). Conceptual challenges and directions for social neuroscience. *Neuron, 65*(6), 752–767.

Agamben, G. (2002). *Remnants of Auschwitz: The witness and the archive* (D. Heller-Roazen, Trans.). New York: Zone Books.

Ahmed, S. (2004). *The cultural politics of emotion*. Edinburgh: Edinburgh University Press.

Albertsen, E., O'Connor, L., & Berry, J. (2006). Religion and interpersonal guilt: Variations across ethnicity and spirituality. *Mental Health, Religion and Culture, 9*(1), 67–84.

Allen, C. (2004). Bourdieu's habitus, social class and the spatial worlds of visually impaired children. *Urban Studies, 41*(3), 487–506.

American Psychiatric Association. (2013). *Diagnostic and statistical manual of mental disorders fifth edition: DSM 5*. Arlington, VA: American Psychiatric Association.

Andersen, S., Reznik, I., & Manzella, L. (1996). Eliciting facial affect, motivation, and expectancies in transference: Significant-other representations in social relations. *Journal of Personality and Social Psychology, 71*(6), 1108–1129.

Anderson, B. (2010). Modulating the excess of affect: Morale in a state of total war. In M. Gregg & G. Seigworth (Eds.), *The Affect Theory Reader* (pp. 161–185). Durham and London: Duke University Press.

Anderson, S. J., Glantz, S. A., & Ling, P. M. (2005). Emotions for sale: Cigarette advertising and women's psychosocial needs. *Tobacco Control, 14*(2), 127–135.

Asbring, P., & Narvanen, A. (2004). Patient power and control: A study of women with uncertain illness trajectories. *Qualitative Health Research, 14*(2), 226–240.

Åsbring, P., & Närvänen, A.-L. (2003). Ideal versus reality: Physicians perspectives on patients with chronic fatigue syndrome (CFS) and fibromyalgia. *Social Science & Medicine, 57*(4), 711–720.

Athanasiou, A., Hantzaroula, P., & Yannakopoulos, Y. (2008). Towards a new epistemology: The 'affective turn'. *Historein, 8*, 5–16.

Atkinson, M. (1984). *Our master's voices: Language and body language of politics*. London: Routledge.

Aukst-Margetic, B., & Margetic, B. (2005). Religiosity and health outcomes: Review of literature. *Collegium Anthropologicum, 29*(1), 365–371.

Azjen, I. (1985). From intentions to actions: A theory of planned behaviour. In J. Kuhl & J. Beckman (Eds.), *Action Control from Cognition to Behaviour* (pp. 11–39). Heidelberg: Springer-Verlag.

Azjen, I., & Fishbein, M. (1980). *Understanding attitudes and predicting social behavior*. Englewood Cliffs, NJ: Prentice Hall.

Baerveldt, C., & Voestermans, P. (2005). Culture, emotion and the normative structure of reality. *Theory and Psychology, 15*(4), 449–474.

Balbach, E., Smith, E., & Malone, R. (2006). How the health belief model helps the tobacco industry: Individuals, choice, and 'information'. *Tobacco Control, 15*(suppl IV), 37–43.

Bamber, D., Craig, O., & Elliott, F. (2003, 16 February 2003). Blair sent in tanks after 'chilling' threat. *The Daily Telegraph*. Retrieved from http://www.telegraph.co.uk/news/uknews/1422243/Blair-sent-in-tanks-after-chilling-threat.html.

Bangert, M., & Altenmueller, E. (2003). Mapping perception to action in piano practice: A longitudinal DC-EEG study. *BMC Neuroscience*. Retrieved 29/11/06, from http://www.pubmedcentral.nih.gov/articlerender.fcgi?artid=270043&tools=bot.

Banks, J., & Prior, L. (2001). Doing things with illness: The micro-politics of the CFS clinic. *Social Science and Medicine, 52*(1), 1–23.

Bar, N., & Ben-Ali, E. (2005). Israeli snipers in the Al-Aqsa intifada: Killing, humanity and lived experience. *Third World Quarterly, 26*(1), 133–152.

Barker, M., Iantaffi, A., & Gupta, C. (2007). Kinky clients, kinky counselling? The challenges and potentials of BDSM. In L. Moon (Ed.), *Feeling Queer or Queer Feelings: Radical Approaches to Counselling Sex, Sexualities and Genders* (pp. 106–124). London: Routledge.

Barlow, J. H., Wright, C. C., Turner, A. P., & Bancroft, G. V. (2005). A 12-month follow-up study of self-management training for people with chronic disease: Are changes maintained over time? *British Journal of Health Psychology, 10*(4), 589–599.

Barnes, T., & Sheppard, E. (1992). Is there a place for the rational actor? A geographical critique of the rational choice paradigm. *Economic Geography, 68*(1), 1–21.

Barrett, L. F. (2006). Solving the emotion paradox: Categorization and the experience of emotion. *Personality and Social Psychology Review, 10*(1), 20–46.

Barsalou, L. W. (1999). Perceptual symbol systems. *Behavioral and Brain Sciences, 22*(04), 577–660.

Barsalou, L., Niedenthal, P., Barbey, A., & Ruppert, J. (2003). Social embodiment. In B. Ross (Ed.), *The Psychology of Learning and Motivation* (pp. 43–92). San Diego: Academic Press.

Barsky, J., & Nash, L. (2002). Evoking emotion: Affective keys to hotel loyalty. *The Cornell Hotel and Restaurant Administration Quarterly, 43*(1), 39–46.

Baumann, Z. (2006). *Liquid fear*. Oxford: Polity Press.

Bechara, A., Damasio, H., Damasio, A. R., & Lee, G. (1999). Different contributions of the human amygdala and ventromedial prefrontal cortex to decision-making. *Journal of Neuroscience, 19*(13), 5473–5481.

Beckmann, A. (2001). Deconstructing myths: The social construction of 'sadomasochism' versus 'subjugated knowledges' of practitioners of consensual 'SM'. *Journal of Criminal Justice and Popular Culture, 8*(2), 66–95.

Bennett, K., & Vidal-Hall, S. (2000). Narratives of death: A qualitative study of widowhood in later life. *Ageing and Society, 20*, 413–428.

Bennett, M. R., & Hacker, P. M. S. (2003). *Philosophical foundations of neuroscience*. Oxford: Blackwells.

Bennett, T., Dodsworth, F., Noble, G., Poovey, M., & Watkins, M. (2013). Habit and Habituation: Governance and the Social. *Body & Society, 19*(2–3), 3–29.

Bentall, R. (2003). *Madness explained*. London: Allen Lane/Penguin.

Bentall, R., & Kaney, S. (2005). Attributional lability in depression and paranoia. *British Journal of Clinical Psychology, 44*, 475–488.

Bentall, R., Corcoran, R., Howard, R., Blackwood, R., & Kinderman, P. (2001). Persecutory delusions: A review and theoretical integration. *Clinical Psychology Review, 21*, 1143–1192.

Billig, M. (1978). *Fascists: A social psychological view of the National Front.* London: Harcourt Bruce Jovanovich.

Billig, M. (1987). *Arguing and thinking: A rhetorical approach to social psychology.* Cambridge: Cambridge University Press.

Billig, M. (1999). *Freudian repression: Conversation creating the unconscious.* Cambridge: Cambridge University Press.

Billig, M., Antaki, C., Butter, C., Cramer, D., Edwards, D., Kent, A., Potter, J., Wilkinson, S., & Tileaga, C. (2011). Benchmarking and social psychology. *The Psychologist, 24*(10), 710–711.

Blackman, L. (2012). *Immaterial bodies: Affect, embodiment, mediation.* London: Sage.

Blackman, L., & Cromby, J. (2007). Affect and feeling. *International Journal of Critical Psychology, 21*, 5–22.

Blackman, L., Cromby, J., Hook, D., Papadopoulos, D., & Walkerdine, V. (2008). Creating subjectivities. *Subjectivity, 22*, 1–27.

Borger, J. (2014, 9 December). US report on 'enhanced interrogation' concludes: Torture doesn't work. *The Guardian.*

Bourdieu, P. (1977). *Outline of a theory of practice* (R. Nice, Trans.). Cambridge: Cambridge University Press.

Bowers, J. (1990). All hail the great abstraction: Star wars and the politics of cognitive psychology. In I. Parker & J. Shotter (Eds.), *Deconstructing Social Psychology* (pp. 127–140). London: Sage Publications.

Boydell, J., Van Os, J., McKenzie, K., Allardyce, J., Goel, R., McCreadie, G., & Murray, R. (2001). Incidence of schizophrenia in ethnic minorities in London: Ecological study into interactions with environment. *British Medical Journal, 323*, 1336–1338.

Boyle, M. (2002). *Schizophrenia: A scientific delusion?* (2nd ed.). London: Routledge.

Bradley, B. (2005). *Psychology and experience.* Cambridge: Cambridge University Press.

Braun, V., & Clarke, V. (2006). Using thematic analysis in psychology. *Qualitative Research in Psychology, 3*, 77–101.

Braun, V., & Clarke, V. (2013). *Successful qualitative research: A practice guide for researchers.* London: Sage Publications.

Brooks-Bouson, J. (2001). 'You nothing but trash': White trash shame in Dorothy Allison's bastard out of Carolina. *Southern Literary Journal, 34*(1), 101–123.

Brooks-Bouson, J. (2005). True confessions: Uncovering the hidden culture of shame in English studies. *JAC, 25*(4), 625–650.

Brown, J. D. (1993). Self-esteem and self-evaluation: Feeling is believing. In J. Suls (Ed.), *Psychological Perspectives on the Self, Volume 4: The Self in Social Perspective* (pp. 27–58). Hove: Psychology Press.

Brown, S. D. (1996). The textuality of stress: Drawing between scientific and everyday accounting. *Journal of Health Psychology, 1*(2), 173–193.

Brown, S. D., & Stenner, P. (2009). *Psychology without foundations: History, philosophy and psychosocial theory.* London: Sage Publications.

Brown, W. (2006). American nightmare: Neoliberalism, neoconservatism and de-democratisation. *Political Theory, 34*(6), 690–714.

Brown, W. J., Basil, M. D., & Bocarnea, M. C. (2003). Social influence of an international celebrity: Responses to the death of princess Diana. *Journal of Communication, 53*(4), 587–605.

Bruner, J., & Goodman, C. C. (1947). Value and need as organising factors in perception. *Journal of Abnormal and Social Psychology, 42*, 33–44.

Bucci, W. (1997). *Psychoanalysis and cognitive science: A multiple code theory.* New York: Guilford Press.

Burkitt, I. (2014). *Emotions and social relations.* London: Sage.

Burston, D. (2014). Humanism. In T. Teo (Ed.), *Encyclopaedia of Critical Psychology* (pp. 915–918). New York: Springer.

Bush, L., Barr, C., McHugo, G., & Lanzetta, J. (1989). The effects of facial control and facial mimicry on subjective reactions to comedy routines. *Motivation and Emotion, 13*(1), 31–52.

Byrne, A. (1994). Behaviourism. Retrieved from http://web.mit.edu/abyrne/www/behaviourism.html.

Byrne, M., Agerbo, E., Eaton, W., & Mortensen, P. (2004). Parental socio-economic status and risk of first admission with schizophrenia. *Social Psychiatry and Psychiatric Epidemiology, 39*(2), 87–96.

Cacioppo, J., Berntson, G., Lorig, T., Norris, C., Rickett, E., & Nusbaum, H. (2003). Just because you're imaging the brain doesn't mean you can stop using your head: A primer and set of first principles. *Journal of Personality and Social Psychology, 85*(4), 650–661.

Cacioppo, J., Priester, J., & Berntson, G. (1993). Rudimentary determinants of attitudes. II: Arm flexion and extension have differential effects on attitudes. *Journal of Personality and Social Psychology, 65*(1), 5–17.

Chakraborty, A., & McKenzie, K. (2002). Does racial discrimination cause mental illness? *British Journal of Psychiatry, 180*, 475–477.

Chalmers, D. (1995). Facing up to the problem of consciousness. *Journal of Consciousness Studies, 2*(3), 200–219.

Chamberlain, K. (2012). Do you really need a methodology? *QMiP Bulletin, 13*, 59–63.

Chamberlain, K., Cain, T., Sheridan, J., & Dupuis, A. (2011). Pluralisms in qualitative research: From multiple methods to integrated methods. *Qualitative Research in Psychology, 8*, 151–169.

Charlesworth, S. (1999). *A phenomenology of working class experience.* Cambridge: Cambridge University Press.

Chida, Y., Steptoe, A., & Powell, L. (2009). Religiosity/spirituality and mortality. *Psychotherapy and Psychosomatics, 78*, 81–90.

Ciompi, L., & Panksepp, J. (2005). Energetic effects of emotions on cognitions: Complementary psychobiological and psychosocial findings. In R. Ellis & N. Newton (Eds.), *Consciousness & Emotion: Agency, Conscious Choice, and Selective Perception* (pp. 23–55). Amsterdam: John Benjamin.

Clark, A. (1998). Embodied, situated, and distributed cognition. In W. Bechtel & G. Graham (Eds.), *A Companion to Cognitive Science* (pp. 506–517). Oxford: Blackwell.

Clark, J., & James, S. (2003). The radicalised self: The impact on the self of the contested nature of the diagnosis of chronic fatigue syndrome. *Social Science and Medicine, 57*, 1387–1395.

Clarke, N. J., Willis, M. E. H., Barnes, J. S., Caddick, N., Cromby, J., McDermott, H., & Wiltshire, G. (2015). Analytical pluralism in qualitative research: A meta-study. *Qualitative Research in Psychology, 12*(2), 182–201.

Clough, P. (2010). Afterword: The future of affect studies. *Body & Society, 16*(1), 222–230.

Clough, P., & Halley, J. (Eds.). (2007). *The affective turn: Theorising the social.* Durham, NC: Duke University Press.

Coates, J., & Herbert, J. (2008). Endogenous steroids and financial risk taking on a London trading floor. *Proceedings of the National Academy of Science (USA).* Retrieved from http://www.pnas.org/cgi/content/abstract/0704025105v1.

Combs, D., Michael, C., & Penn, D. (2006). Paranoia and emotion perception across the continuum. *British Journal of Clinical Psychology, 45*, 19–31.

Connolly, W. (2002). *Neuropolitics: Thinking, culture, speed.* Minneapolis: University of Minnesota Press.

Corcoran, T. (2009). Second nature. *British Journal of Social Psychology, 48*(2), 375–388.

Cox, T. (2014). *Sonic Wonderland: A scientific Odyssey of sound.* Oxford: Bodley Head.

Crawford, J., Kippax, S., Onyx, J., Gault, U., & Benton, P. (1992). *Emotion and gender: Constructing meaning from memory.* London: Sage Publications.

Cromby, J. (2007a). Integrating social science with neuroscience: Potentials and problems. *Biosocieties, 2*(2), 149–170.

Cromby, J. (2007b). Toward a psychology of feeling. *International Journal of Critical Psychology, 21*, 94–118. Retrieved from http://www.johncromby.webspace.virginmedia.com/.

Cromby, J. (2011). The greatest gift? Happiness, governance and psychology. *Social and Personality Psychology Compass, 5*(11), 840–852.

Cromby, J. (2012). Response to commentaries on 'Beyond Belief'. *Journal of Health Psychology, 17*(7), 982–988.

Cromby, J. (2015). The public meanings of CFS/ME: Making up people. In C. Ward (Ed.), *Meanings of ME: Interpersonal and Social Dimensions of Chronic Fatigue.* London: Palgrave.

Cromby, J., Brown, S. D., Gross, H., Locke, A., & Patterson, A. E. (2010). Constructing crime, enacting morality: Emotion, crime and anti-social behaviour in an inner-city community. *British Journal of Criminology, 50*(5), 873–895.

Cromby, J., & Harper, D. (2009). Paranoia: A social account. *Theory and Psychology, 19*(3), 335–361.

Cromby, J., Harper, D., & Reavey, P. (2013). *Psychology, mental health and distress.* London: Palgrave.

Cromby, J., Harper, D., & Sutton, N. (2006). *Paranoia, Social Inequality and Feelings.* Paper presented at the International Conference on Qualitative Research and Marginalisation.

Cromby, J., & Nightingale, D. J. (1999). What's wrong with social constructionism? In D. J. Nightingale & J. Cromby (Eds.), *Social Constructionist Psychology: A Critical Analysis of Theory and Practice* (pp. 1–20). Buckingham: Open University Press.

Cromby, J., & Phillips, A. (2014). Feeling bodies: Analysing the unspeakability of death. In L. van Brussel & N. Carpentier (Eds.), *The Social Construction of Death: Interdisciplinary Perspectives* (pp. 52–74). London: Palgrave.

Cromby, J., & Willis, M. E. H. (2014). Nudging into subjectification: Governmentality and psychometrics. *Critical Social Policy, 34*(2), 241–259.

Cromby, J., Harper, D., & Reavey, P. (2013). *Psychology, Mental Health and Distress.* London: Palgrave.

Cromby, J., Harper, D., & Sutton, N. (2006). Paranoia, Social Inequality and Feelings. Paper presented at the International Conference on Qualitative Research and Marginalisation.

Cusick, S. G. (2006). Music as torture/music as weapon. *Transcultural Music Review, 10, 39.*

Cusick, S. G. (2008). 'You are in a place that is out of the world...': Music in the detention camps of the 'Global War on Terror'. *Journal of the Society for American Music, 2*(01), 1–26.

Damasio, A. R. (1994). *Descartes error: Emotion, reason and the human brain.* London: Picador.

Damasio, A. R. (1999). *The feeling of what happens: Body, emotion and the making of consciousness.* London: William Heinemann.

Danziger, K. (1994). *Constructing the subject: Historical origins of psychological research.* Cambridge: Cambridge University Press.

Darker, C., & French, D. (2009). What sense do people make of a theory of planned behaviour questionnaire? A think-aloud study. *Journal of Health Psychology, 14,* 861–871.

Davies, C. (2012). Rite out of time: A study of the churching of women and its survival in the twentieth century. *Journal of Contemporary Religion, 27*(2), 340–341.

Day, A. (2010). Propositions and performativity: Relocating belief to the social. *Culture and Religion, 11*(1), 9–30.

Day, A., & Coleman, S. (2010). Broadening boundaries: Creating interdisciplinary dialogue on belief. *Culture and Religion, 11*(1), 1–8.

Dimberg, U., Thunberg, M., & Elmehed, K. (2000). Unconscious facial reactions to emotional facial expressions. *Psychological Science, 11*(1), 86–89.

Dinos, S., Stevens, S., Serfaty, M., Weich, S., & King, M. (2004). Stigma: The feelings and experiences of 46 people with mental illness: Qualitative study. *The British Journal of Psychiatry, 184*(2), 176–181.

Dixon, T. (2003). *From passions to emotions: The creation of a secular psychological category.* Cambridge: Cambridge University Press.

Dohrenwend, B. S., & Dohrenwend, B. P. (Eds.). (1974). *Stressful life events: Their nature and effects.* New York: John Wiley.

Double, D. (Ed.). (2006). *Critical psychiatry: The limits of madness.* Basingstoke: Palgrave.

Downing, L. (2012). Safewording! kinkphobia and gender normativity in fifty shades of grey. *Psychology & Sexuality, 4*(1), 92–102.

Duff, K. (2003). Social effects of chronic disorders. In L. A. Jason, P. A. Fennell & R. R. Taylor (Eds.), *Handbook of Chronic Fatigue Syndrome* (pp. 176–191). Hoboken, NJ: John Wiley.

Dumit, J. (2004). *Picturing personhood: Brain scans and biomedical identity.* Princeton, NJ: Princeton University Press.

Duncan, S., & Barrett, L. F. (2007). Affect is a form of cognition: A neurobiological analysis. *Cognition and Emotion, 21*(6), 1184–1211.

Durkheim, E. (1995 [1912]). *The elementary forms of religious life.* New York: Free Press.

Eaton, L. (2002). A third of Europeans and almost half of Americans use internet for health information. *British Medical Journal, 325*, 989.

Eatough, V., & Smith, J. (2006). 'I was like a wild wild person': Understanding feelings of anger using interpretative phenomenological analysis. *British Journal of Psychology, 97*(4), 483–498.

Edley, N., & Wetherell, M. (1995). *Men in perspective: Practice, power and identity.* London: Prentice Hall/Harvester Wheatsheaf.

Edwards, D. (1997). *Discourse and cognition.* London: Sage Publications.

Edwards, D. (1999). Emotion discourse. *Culture and Psychology, 5*(3), 271–291.

Edwards, D., & Potter, J. (1992). *Discursive psychology.* London: Sage Publications.

Ehrenreich, B. (2007). *Dancing in the streets: A history of collective joy.* London: Granta.

Ekman, P. (1992). Are there basic emotions? *Psychological Review, 99*(3), 550–553.

Ellis, D., & Tucker, I. (2011). Virtuality and Ernest Bloch: Hope and subjectivity. *Subjectivity, 4*(4), 434–450.

Ellis, D., Tucker, I., & Harper, D. (2013). The affective atmospheres of surveillance. *Theory & Psychology, 23*(6), 716–731.

England, P. (1989). A feminist critique of rational-choice theories: Implications for sociology. *The American Sociologist, 20*(1), 14–28.

Evaldsson, A.-C. (2003). Throwing like a girl? Situating gender differences in physicality across game contexts. *Childhood, 10*(4), 475–497.

Evans, S., Tsao, J. C. I., Lu, Q., Myers, C., Suresh, J., & Zeltzer, L. K. (2008). Parent-child pain relationships from a psychosocial perspective: A review of the literature. *Journal of Pain Management, 1*(3), 237–246.

Everson-Rose, S., & Lewis, T. (2005). Psychosocial factors and cardiovascular diseases. *Annual Review of Public Health, 26*, 469–500.

Falmagne, R. J. (2012). Leaving dualisms behind: Felt thinking and the social. Commentary of John Cromby, 'Beyond belief'. *Journal of Health Psychology, 17*(7), 962–964.

Feinstein, J., Goldin, P., Stein, M., Brown, G., & Paulus, M. (2002). Habituation of attentional networks during emotion processing. *Neuroreport, 13*(10), 1255–1258.

Fennell, P. A. (2003). Sociocultural context and trauma. In L. A. Jason, P. A. Fennell & R. R. Taylor (Eds.), *Handbook of Chronic Fatigue Syndrome* (pp. 73–88). Hoboken, NJ: John Wiley.

Findley, J., Kerns, R., Weinberg, L., & Rosenberg, R. (1998). Self-efficacy as a psychological moderator of chronic fatigue syndrome. *Journal of Behavioral Medicine, 21*(4), 351–362.

Focht, B., Bouchard, L., & Murphey, M. (2000). Influence of martial arts training on the perception of experimentally induced pressure pain and selected psychological responses. *Journal of Sport Behaviour, 23*, 232–244.

Forster, J., & Strack, F. (1996). Influence of overt head movements on memory for valenced words: A case of conceptual-motor compatibility. *Journal of Personality and Social Psychology, 71*(3), 421–430.

Fox, D., Prilletensky, I., & Austin, S. (2009). *Critical psychology: An introduction.* London: Sage Publications.

Fox, E. (2008). *Emotion science*. London: Palgrave Macmillan.

Francis, L. J. (1993). Reliability and validity of a short scale of attitude towards Christianity among adults. *Psychological Reports, 72*, 615–618.

Franklin, L. (2011). *Parenting in the culture of fear*. Loughborough: Loughborough University.

Fredrickson, B. L., & Harrison, K. (2005). Throwing like a girl: Self-objectification predicts adolescent girls' motor performance. *Journal of Sport & Social Issues, 29*(1), 79–101.

Freeman, D., Garety, P. A., Kuipers, E., Fowler, D., & Bebbington, P. (2002). A cognitive model of persecutory delusions. *British Journal of Clinical Psychology, 41*, 331–347.

Frijda, N. (1988). The laws of emotion. *American Psychologist, 43*(5), 349–358.

Furedi, F. (2007). *Culture of fear revisited*. London: Continuum.

Fyson, R., & Cromby, J. (2013). Human rights and intellectual disabilities in an era of 'choice'. *Journal of Intellectual Disability Research, 57*(12), 1164–1172.

Galvin, R. (2002). Disturbing notions of chronic illness and individual responsibility: Towards a genealogy of morals. *Health, 6*(2), 107–137.

Gardner, H. (1985). *The mind's new science: A history of the cognitive revolution*. New York: Basic Books.

Garety, P. A. (1985). Delusions: Problems in definition and measurement. *British Journal of Medical Psychology, 58*, 25–34.

Geelen, S., Sinnema, G., Hermans, H., & Kuis, W. (2007). Personality and chronic fatigue syndrome: Methodological and conceptual issues. *Clinical Psychology Review, 27*, 885–903.

Georgaca, E. (2004). Factualization and plausibility in 'delusional' discourse. *Philosophy, Psychiatry and Psychology, 11*, 13–23.

Gerberhagen, K., Trojan, M., Kuhn, J., Limroth, V., & Bewermeyer, H. (2008). Significance of health-related quality of life and religiosity for the acceptance of chronic pain. *Schmerz, 22*(5), 586–593.

Gier, N. F. (1976). Intentionality and prehension. *Process Studies, 6*(3), 197–213.

Gill, R. C. (2009). Secrecy, silence, toxic shame and the hidden injuries of the neo-liberal university. In R. C. Gill & R. Ryan-Flood (Eds.), *Secrecy and Silence in the Research Process: Feminist Reflections* (pp. 228–244). London: Routledge.

Gillham, B., Tanner, G., Cheyne, B., Freeman, I., Rooney, M., & Lambie, A. (1998). Uemployment rates, single parent density, and indices of child poverty: Their relationship to different categories of child abuse and neglect. *Child Abuse and Neglect, 22*(2), 79–90.

Gillies, V., Harden, A., Johnson, K., Reavey, P., Strange, V., & Willig, C. (2004). Women's collective constructions of embodied practices through memory work: An exploration of memories of sweating and pain. *British Journal of Social Psychology, 43*, 99–112.

Gillies, V., Harden, A., Johnson, K., Reavey, P., Strange, V., & Willig, C. (2005). Painting pictures of embodied experience: The use of non-linguistic data in the study of embodiment. *Qualitative Research in Psychology, 2*(3), 199–212.

Glassner, B. (1999). *The culture of fear: Why Americans are afraid of the wrong things*. New York: Basic Books.

Goodin, R. E., & Saward, M. (2005). Dog whistles and democratic mandates. *The Political Quarterly, 76*(4), 471–476.

Goodman, S. (2012). *Sonic warfare: Sound, affect and the ecology of fear*. Cambridge, MA: M.I.T. Press.

Goudsmit, E. M., Nijs, J., Jason, L. A., & Wallman, K. E. (2012). Pacing as a strategy to improve energy management in myalgic encephalomyelitis/chronic fatigue syndrome: A consensus document. *Disability and Rehabilitation, 34*(13), 1140–1147.

Graham, H. (1987). Women's smoking and family health. *Social Science & Medicine, 25*(1), 47–56.

Green, D., & Shapiro, I. (1994). The nature of rational choice. In D. Green & I. Shapiro (Eds.), *Pathologies of Rational Choice Theory* (pp. 13–32). New Haven: Yale University Press.

Greenwald, G. (2014). *No place to hide: Edward snowden, the NSA and the surveillance state*. London: Hamish Hamilton.

Gregg, M., & Seigworth, G. (Eds.). (2010). *The affect theory reader*. Durham and London: Duke University Press.

Griffiths, P. (1998). *What emotions really are: The problem of psychological categories*. Chicago: University of Chicago Press.

Grossberg, L. (1992). *We gotta get out of this place*. London: Routledge.

Guise, J., Widdicombe, S., & McKinlay, A. (2007). 'What is it like to have ME?': The discursive construction of ME in computer-mediated communication and face-to-face interaction. *Health, 11*(1), 87–108.

Gunnar, M., & Donzella, B. (2002). Social regulation of the cortisol levels in early human development. *Psychoneuroendocrinology, 27*, 199–220.

Ha, H.-Y., & Perks, H. (2005). Effects of consumer perceptions of brand experience on the web: Brand familiarity, satisfaction and brand trust. *Journal of Consumer Behaviour, 4*(6), 438–452.

Hacking, I. (2006, 17 August). Making up people. *London Review of Books, 28*(16), 23–26.

Hagger, M., & Chatzisarantis, N. (2009). Integrating the theory of planned behaviour and self-determination theory in health behaviour: A meta-analysis. *British Journal of Health Psychology, 14*(2), 275–302.

Haraway, D. (1996). *Simians, cyborgs and women: The reinvention of nature*. New York: Free Association Books.

Hardt, M. (1999). Affective labour. *Boundary 2, 26*(2), 89–100.

Harper, D. (2004). Delusions and discourse: Moving beyond the constraints of the rationalist paradigm. *Philosophy, Psychiatry and Psychology, 11*, 55–64.

Harre, R. (Ed.). (1986). *The social construction of emotion*. Oxford: Blackwells.

Harre, R. (1992). The second cognitive revolution. *American Behavioural Scientist, 36*, 3–7.

Harre, R. (1999). Discourse and the embodied person. In D. J. Nightingale & J. Cromby (Eds.), *Social Constructionist Psychology: A Critical Analysis of Theory and Practice* (pp. 97–112). Buckingham: Open University Press.

Harre, R. (2002). *Cognitive science: A philosophical introduction*. London: Sage Publications.

Harrison, G., Gunnell, D., Glazebrook, C., Page, K., & Kwiecinski, R. (2001). Association between schizophrenia and social inequality at birth: Case-control study. *British Journal of Psychiatry, 179*, 346–350.

Harrop, C., & Trower, P. (2003). *Why does schizophrenia develop at late adolescence?: A cognitive-developmental approach to psychosis*. Chichester: Wiley.

Haug, F. (1987). *Female sexualisation: A collective work of memory* (E. Carter, Trans.). London: Verso.

Healy, D. (1987). Rhythm and blues: Neurochemical, neuropharmacological and neuropsychological implications of a hypothesis of circadian rhythm dysfunction in the affective disorders. *Psychopharmacology, 93,* 271–285.

Hemmings, C. (2005). Invoking affect: Cultural theory and the ontological turn. *Cultural Studies, 19*(5), 548–567.

Hepburn, A., & Wiggins, S. (2005). Developments in discursive psychology. *Discourse and Society, 16*(5), 595–601.

Herman, J. (2007). *Shattered Shame States and their Repair.* Paper presented at the The John Bowlby Memorial Lecture, London

Hermans, H. (2002). The dialogical self as a society of mind. *Theory and Psychology, 12*(2), 147–160.

Highmore, B. (2010). Bitter after taste. In M. Gregg & G. Seigworth (Eds.), *The Affect Theory Reader* (pp. 118–137). Durham and London: Duke University Press.

Hiller, J. (2005). Sex, mind and emotion through the life course: A biopsychosocial perspective. In J. Hiller, H. Wood & W. Bolton (Eds.), *Sex, Mind and Emotion* (pp. 3–40). London: Karnac.

Hochschild, A. R. (1983). *The managed heart: The commercialisation of human feeling.* Berkeley: University of California Press.

Hoffman, R., Cochran, E., & Nead, J. (1990). Cognitive metaphors in the history of experimental psychology. In D. Leary (Ed.), *Metaphors in the History of Psychology* (pp. 173–209). Cambridge: Cambridge University Press.

Honderich, T. (Ed.). (1995). *The oxford companion to philosophy.* Oxford: Oxford University Press.

Hook, D. (2007). *Foucault, psychology and the analytics of power.* London: Palgrave.

Horton-Salway, M. (2001). Narrative identities and the management of personal accountability in talk about ME: A discursive psychology approach to illness narrative. *Journal of Health Psychology, 6*(2), 247–259.

Horton-Salway, M. (2004). The local production of knowledge: Disease labels, identities and category entitlements in ME support group talk. *Health, 8*(3), 351–371.

Houdenhove, B. v., & Luyten, P. (2008). Customizing treatment of chronic fatigue syndrome and fibromyalgia: The role of perpetuating factors. *Psychosomatics, 49*(6), 470–477.

Hui, C. H., & Triandis, H. C. (1986). Individualism-collectivism: A study of cross-cultural researchers. *Journal of Cross-Cultural Psychology, 17*(2), 225–248.

Hyland, K. (1996). Writing without conviction? Hedging in science research articles. *Applied Linguistics, 17*(4), 433–454.

Hyland, M. (2002). The intelligent body and its discontents. *Journal of Health Psychology, 7*(1), 21–32.

Illousz, E. (2012). *Cold intimacies: The making of emotional capitalism.* Cambridge: Polity Press.

Innis, R. (2009). *Susanne Langer in focus: The symbolic mind.* Bloomington: Indiana University Press.

Jack, G. (2004). Child protection at the community level. *Child Abuse Review, 13,* 368–383.

Jacobson, N., & Truax, P. (1991). Clinical significance: A statistical approach to defining meaningful change in psychotherapy research. *Journal of Consulting and Clinical Psychology, 59*(1), 12–19.

Jaggar, A. (1989). Love and knowledge: Emotion in feminist epistemology. *Inquiry, 32*, 151–172.

James, W. (1892). The stream of consciousness, from *Psychology*. Retrieved 25/01/06, from http://psychclassics.yorku.ca/James/jimmy11.html.

Jansen, A., Smeets, T., Martijn, C., & Nederkoorn, C. (2006). I see what you see: The lack of a self-serving body-image bias in eating disorders. *British Journal of Clinical Psychology, 45*, 123–135.

Jason, L. A., Taylor, R. R., Stepanek, Z., & Plioplys, S. (2001). Attitudes regarding chronic fatigue syndrome: The importance of a name. *Journal of Health Psychology, 6*(1), 61–71.

Jervis, R. (2006). Understanding beliefs. *Political Psychology, 27*(5), 641–663.

Johns, L. C., Cannon, M., Singleton, N., Murray, R. M., Farrell, M., Brugha, T., Bebbington, P., Jenkins, R., & Meltzer, H. (2004). Prevalence and correlates of self-reported psychotic symptoms in the British population. *British Journal of Psychiatry, 185*, 298–305.

Johnson, M. (2007). *The meaning of the body: Aesthetics of human understanding.* Chicago: University of Chicago Press.

Johnson, M., Long, T., & White, A. (2000). Arguments for 'British Pluralism' in qualitative health research. *Journal of Advanced Nursing, 33*(2), 243–249.

Johnstone, L. (2000). *Users and abusers of psychiatry* (2nd ed.). Hove: Brunner-Routledge.

Jones, D., & Elcock, J. (2001). *History and theories of psychology: A critical perspective.* London: Arnold (Hodder Headline).

Jones, N., Field, T., Fox, N., Davalos, M., & Malphus, J. (1997). Infants of intrusive and withdrawn mothers. *Infant Behaviour and Development, 20*, 175–186.

Jones, R., Pykett, J., & Whitehead, M. (2013). *Changing behaviours: On the rise of the psychological state.* Cheltenham: Edward Elgar Publishing Ltd.

Kagan, J. (1998). *Three seductive ideas.* Cambridge, MA: Harvard University Press.

Kahneman, D. (2012). *Thinking fast and slow.* London: Penguin.

Kahneman, D., Krueger, A., Schkade, D., Schwarz, N., & Stone, A. (2004). A survey method for characterising daily life experience: The day reconstruction method. *Science, 306*(5702), 1776–1780.

Karademas, E. (2010). Illness cognitions as a pathway between religiousness and subjective health in chronic cardiac patients. *Journal of Health Psychology, 15*, 239–247.

Kendler, K. S. (1982). Demography of paranoid psychosis (delusional disorder): A review and comparison with schizophrenia and affective illness. *Archives of General Psychiatry, 39*, 890–902.

Khalliatt, M. (2013). *Beneath the anthropomorphic veil: Animal imagery and ideological discourses in British advertising.* London: LSE.

Kiecolt-Glaser, J., McGuire, L., Robles, T., & Glaser, R. (2002). Psychoneuroimmunology: Psychological influences on immune function and health. *Journal of Consulting and Clinical Psychology, 70*, 537–547.

Kincheloe, J., & Berry, K. (2004). *Rigour and complexity in educational research: Conceptualising the bricolage.* Maidenhead: Open University Press.

King, M., Coker, E., Leavey, A., Hoare, A., & Johnson-Sabine, D. (1994). Incidence of psychotic illness in London: Comparison of ethnic groups. *British Medical Journal, 309*, 1115–1119.

Kiser, E., & Hechter, M. (1998). The debate on historical sociology: Rational choice theory and its critics. *American Journal of Sociology, 104*(3), 785–816.

Knoop, H., Prins, J., Moss-Morris, R., & Bleijenberg, G. (2010). The central role of cognitive processes in the perpetuation of chronic fatigue syndrome. *Journal of Psychosomatic Research, 68*, 489–494.

Koenig, H. G., Cohen, H., George, L., Hays, J., Larson, D. B., & Blazer, D. (1997). Attendance at religious services, interleukin-6, and other biological parameters of immune function in older adults. *International Journal of Psychiatry in Medicine, 27*, 233–250.

Koenig, H. G., McCullough, M. E., & Larson, D. B. (2000). *Handbook of religion and health.* New York: Oxford University Press.

Kohn, L. (1976). The interaction of social class and other factors in the etiology of schizophrenia. *American Journal of Psychiatry, 133*(2), 177–180.

Kühberger, A., Fritz, A., & Scherndl, T. (2014). Publication bias in psychology: A diagnosis based on the correlation between effect size and sample size. *PLoS ONE, 9*(9), e105825.

Laing, R. D. (1960). *The divided self: An existential study in sanity and madness.* Harmondsworth: Penguin.

Langdridge, D., & Barker, M. (2007). *Safe, sane and consensual: Contemporary perspectives on sadomasochism.* London: Palgrave.

Langer, S. (1967). *Mind: An essay on human feeling* (Vol. 1). Baltimore: The Johns Hopkins University Press.

Langer, S. (1972). *Mind: An essay on human feeling* (Vol. 2). Baltimore: The Johns Hopkins University Press.

Langer, S. (1982). *Mind: An essay on human feeling* (Vol. 3). Baltimore: The Johns Hopkins University Press.

Lazarus, R. (1982). Thoughts on the relationship between emotion and cognition. *American Psychologist, 37*, 1019–1024.

Leary, D. (1994). *Metaphors in the history of psychology.* Cambridge: Cambridge University Press.

Leder, D. (1990). *The absent body.* Chicago: University of Chicago Press.

Lee, S. (2001). Fat phobia in anorexia: Who obsession is it? In M. Nasser, M. A. Katzman & R. A. Gordon (Eds.), *Eating Disorders and Cultures in Transition* (pp. 40–54). London: Routledge.

Lemert, E. (1962). Paranoia and the dynamics of exclusion. *Sociometry, 25*, 2–20.

Lewis, H. B. (1971). *Shame and guilt in neurosis.* New York: International Universities Press.

Lewis, M. (2002). The dialogical brain: Contributions of emotional neurobiology to understanding the dialogical self. *Theory and Psychology, 12*(2), 175–190.

Leys, R. (2007). *From guilt to shame: Auschwitz and after.* Princeton, NJ: Princeton University Press.

Leys, R. (2011). The turn to affect: A critique. *Critical Inquiry, 37* (Spring 2011), 434–472.

Libet, B. (1993). The neural time – Factor in perception, volition and free will. *Neurophysiology of Consciousness* (pp. 367–384). Boston: Birkhäuser. Retrieved from http://link.springer.com/chapter/10.1007%2F978-1-4612-0355-1_22

Lifton, R. J. (1986). *The Nazi doctors: Medical killing and the psychology of genocide.* New York: Basic Books.

Lindemann, D. (2011). BDSM as therapy? *Sexualities, 14*(2), 151–172.

Lissoni, P., Cangemi, P., Pirato, D., Grazia-Roselli, M., Rovelli, F., Brivio, F., Malugani, F., Maestroni, G., Conti, A., Laudon, M., Malysheva, O., & Giani, L. (2001). A review on cancer-psychospiritual status interactions. *Neuroendocrinology Letters, 22,* 175–180.

Locke, J. L., & Fehr, F. S. (1970). Subvocal rehearsal as a form of speech. *Journal of Verbal Learning and Verbal Behavior, 9*(5), 495–498.

Lorenz, C. (2012). If you're so smart, why are you under surveillance? Universities, neoliberalism and new public management. *Critical Inquiry, 38*(3), 599–629.

Lutz, C. (1988). *Unnatural emotions: Everyday sentiments on a Micronesian Atoll.* Chicago: University of Chicago Press.

Macey, D. (2009). Rethinking biopolitics, race and power in the wake of Foucault. *Theory, Culture and Society, 26*(6), 186–205.

Madill, A., Jordan, A., & Shirley, C. (2000). Objectivity and reliability in qualitative analysis: Realist, contextualist and radical constructionist epistemologies. *British Journal of Psychology, 91,* 1–20.

Maguire, E., Gadian, D., Johnsrude, I., Good, C., Ashburner, J., Frackowiak, R., & Frith, C. (2000). Navigation related structural change in the hippocampi of taxi drivers. *Proceedings of the National Academy of Science (USA), 97*(8), 4398–4403.

Manteufel, A. (2005). Chromosomen non est omen: On the relationship between neurobiology and psychotherapy. *Journal of Systemic Therapies, 24*(3), 70–88.

Marks, D. (2008). The quest for meaningful theory in health psychology. *Journal of Health Psychology, 13,* 977–981.

Marshall, D. (2002). Behaviour, belief and belonging: A theory of ritual practice. *Sociological Theory, 20*(3), 360–380.

Martocci, L. (2015. *Bullying: The social destruction of self.* Philadelphia: Temple University Press.

Massumi, B. (2002). *Parables for the virtual: Movement, affect, sensation.* Durham, NC: Duke University Press.

Massumi, B. (2010). The future birth of the affective fact: The political ontology of threat. In M. Gregg & G. Seigworth (Eds.), *The Affect Theory Reader* (pp. 52–70). Durham and London: Duke University Press.

Mateus, M., Silva, C., Neves, O., & Redondo, J. (2008). Feeders: Eating or sexual disorder? *European Psychiatry, 23,* S184–S185.

McAvoy, J. (2015). From ideology to feeling: Discourse, emotion, and an analytic synthesis. *Qualitative Research in Psychology, 12*(1), 22–33.

McCullough, M. E., Hoyt, W., Larson, D. B., Koenig, H. G., & Thoresen, C. (2000). Religious involvement and mortality: A meta-analytic review. *Health Psychology, 19*(3), 211–222.

McEachan, R., Conner, M., Taylor, N., & Lawton, R. (2011). Prospective prediction of health-related behaviours with the theory of planned behaviour: A meta-analysis. *Health Psychology Review, 5,* 97–114.

McGrath, L., & Reavey, P. (2015). Seeking fluid possibility and solid ground: Space and movement in mental health service users' experiences of 'crisis'. *Social Science & Medicine, 128,* 115–125.

McKenzie, L. (2015). *Getting by: Estates, class and culture in austerity Britain.* Bristol: Policy Press.

McKie, R. (2001, 11 February). Revealed: The secret of human behaviour. *The Observer.*

Meier, B., Schnall, S., Schwarz, N., & Bargh, J. (2012). Embodiment in social psychology. *Topics in Cognitive Science, 4*(4), 705–716.

Meisenhelder, J., & Chandler, E. (2002). Spirituality and health outcomes in the elderly. *Journal of Religion and Health, 41,* 243–252.

Merleau-Ponty, M. (2002). *Phenomenology of perception* (C. Smith, Trans.). London: Routledge.

Meshcheryakov, B. (2007). Terminology in L. S. Vygotsky's writings. In H. Daniels, M. Cole & J. Wertsch (Eds.), *The Cambridge Companion to Vygotsky* (pp. 155–177). Cambridge: Cambridge University Press.

Meyer, C., Waller, G., & Waters, A. (1998). Emotional states and bulimic psychopathology. In H. Hock, J. Treasure & M. Katzman (Eds.), *Neurobiology in the Treatment of Nervous Disorders* (pp. 271–289). London: John Wiley & Sons Ltd.

Michell, J. (2000). Normal science, pathological science and psychometrics. *Theory and Psychology, 10*(5), 639–667.

Middleton, D., & Brown, S. D. (2005). *The social psychology of experience: Studies in remembering and forgetting.* London: Sage Publications.

Mielewczyk, F., & Willig, C. (2007). Old clothes and an older look: The case for a radical makeover in health behaviour. *Theory and Psychology, 17*(6), 811–837.

Millington, B., & Nelson, R. (1986). *Boys from the blackstuff: The making of TV drama.* London: Routledge.

Mitchell, S. A., & Black, M. J. (1995). *Freud and beyond: A history of modern psychoanalytic thought.* New York: Basic Books.

Moloney, P. (2013). *The therapy industry.* London: Pluto Press.

Monaghan, L. (2005). Big handsome men, bears and others: Virtual constructions of 'Fat Male Embodiment'. *Body and Society, 11*(2), 81–111.

Moncrieff, J. (2008). *The myth of the chemical cure: A critique of psychiatric drug treatment.* London: Palgrave.

Morawski, J. (1998). The return of phantom subjects. In B. M. Bayer & J. Shotter (Eds.), *Reconstructing the Psychological Subject* (pp. 214–228). London: Sage Publications.

Morrison, A. P., Frame, L., & Larkin, W. (2003). Relationships between trauma and psychosis: A review and integration. *British Journal of Clinical Psychology, 42,* 331–353.

Mulhall, A. (1996). Cultural discourse and the myth of stress in nursing and medicine. *International Journal of Nursing Studies, 33*(5), 455–468.

Mutch, A. (2003). Communities of practice and habitus: A critique. *Organization Studies, 24*(3), 383–401.

National Institute for Clinical Excellence. (2007). *Chronic fatigue syndrome/myalgic encephalomyelitis (or encephalopathy). Diagnosis and management of CFS/ME in adults and children.* London: National Institute for Health and Clinical Excellence.

Newton, T. (2003). Truly embodied sociology: Marrying the social and the biological. *The Sociological Review, 51*(1), 20–42.

Newton, T. (2007). *Nature and sociology.* London: Routledge.

Norton-Taylor, R. (2015, 12 January). Charlie hebdo, Europe, Britain, and terrorism: Dangers ahead. *The Guardian.*

Ogarkova, A., Soriano, C., & Lehr, C. (2012). Naming feeling: Exploring the equivalence of emotion terms in five European languages. *Lodz Studies in Language, 27*, 253–284.

Ohman, A., Flykt, A., & Esteves, F. (2001). Emotion drives attention: Detecting the snake in the grass. *Journal of Experimental Psychology: General, 130*(3), 466–478.

Olson, G. (2012). *Empathy imperiled: Capitalism, culture, and the brain*. New York: Springer.

Oncken, C., McKee, S., Krishnan-Sarin, S., O'Malley, S., & Mazure, C. M. (2005). Knowledge and perceived risk of smoking-related conditions: A survey of cigarette smokers. *Preventive Medicine, 40*(6), 779–784.

Orlov, A. (2010). *A simples life: The life and times of Aleksandr Orlov*. London: Ebury Press.

Papadopoulos, D. (1996). Observations on Vygotsky's reception in academic psychology. In C. Tolman, F. Cherry, R. van Hezewijk & I. Lubek (Eds.), *Problems of Theoretical Psychology* (pp. 145–155). Toronto: Captus University Press.

Park, C. (2007). Religiousness/spirituality and health: A meaning-systems perspective. *Journal of Behavioural Medicine, 30*, 319–328.

Parker, I. (1989). *The crisis in modern social psychology and how to end it*. London: Routledge.

Parker, I. (1997). *Psychoanalytic culture*. London: Sage Publications.

Parker, I. (2004). Criteria for qualitative research in psychology. *Qualitative Research in Psychology, 1*, 1–12.

Parker, I. (2014). Austerity in the university. *The Psychologist, 27*, 236–239.

Parker, I. (2015). Walls and holes in psychosocial research: From psychoanalysis to critique. *Qualitative Research in Psychology, 12*(1), 77–82.

Pashler, H., & Wagenmakers, E. (2012). Editors' introduction to the special section on replicability in psychological science: A crisis of confidence? *Perspectives on Psychological Science, 7*(6), 528–530.

Patterson, A., Khogeer, Y., & Hodgson, J. (2012). How to create an influential anthropomorphic mascot: Literary musings on marketing, make-believe, and meerkats. *Journal of Marketing Management, 29*(1–2), 69–85.

Phelps, E. A. (2006). Emotion and cognition: Insights from studies of the human amygdala. *Annual Review of Psychology, 57*(1), 27–53.

Phillips, A. (1994). *On kissing, tickling and being bored: Psychoanalyic essays on the unexamined life*. London: Faber and Faber.

Phoenix, C., & Orr, N. (2014). Pleasure: A forgotten dimension of activity in older age. *Social Science & Medicine, 115*, 94–102.

Pieslak, J. R. (2007). Sound targets: Music and the war in Iraq. *Journal of Musicological Research, 26*(2–3), 123–149.

Pitts-Taylor, V. (2010). The plastic brain: Neoliberalism and the neuronal self. *Health, 14*(6), 635–652.

Potter, J. (1996). *Representing reality: Discourse, rhetoric and social construction*. London: Sage Publications.

Potter, J., & Hepburn, A. (2005). Qualitative interviews in psychology: Problems and possibilities. *Qualitative Research in Psychology, 2*, 1–27.

Potter, J., & Wetherell, M. (1987). *Discourse and social psychology: Beyond attitudes and behaviour*. London: Sage Publications.

Pressman, S., & Cohen, S. (2005). Does positive affect influence health? *Psychological Bulletin, 131*(5), 925–971.

Prinz, J. (2004). *Gut reactions: A perceptual theory of emotion*. New York: Oxford University Press.

Probyn, E. (2004). Everyday shame. *Cultural Studies, 18*(2–3), 328–349.

Radley, A., & Taylor, D. (2003). Images of recovery: A photo-elicitation study on the hospital ward. *Qualitative Health Research, 13*(1), 77–99.

Ratner, C. (2000). A cultural-psychological analysis of emotions. *Culture and Psychology, 6*, 5–39.

Ray, L. (2014). Shame and the city – 'looting', emotions and social structure. *The Sociological Review, 62*, 117–136.

Read, J. (2009). A genealogy of homo-economicus: Neoliberalism and the production of subjectivity. *Foucault Studies, 6*, 25–36.

Read, J., van Os, J., Morrison, A. P., & Ross, C. A. (2005). Childhood trauma, psychosis and schizophrenia: A literature review with theoretical and clinical implications. *Acta-Psychiatrica-Scandinavica, 112*, 330–350.

Reavey, P. (Ed.). (2011). *Visual methods in psychology: Using and interpreting images in qualitative research*. Hove: Psychology Press.

Reavey, P., & Johnson, K. (2008). Visual approaches: Using and interpreting images. In C. Willig & W. Stainton-Rogers (Eds.), *The Sage Handbook of Qualitative Research in Psychology* (pp. 296–314). London: Sage Publications.

Rew, L., & Wong, Y. (2006). A systematic review of associations between religiosity/spirituality and adolescent health attitudes and behaviours. *Journal of Adolescent Health, 38*, 433–442.

Rhudy, J., Williams, A., McCabe, K., Rambo, P., & Russell, J. (2006). Emotional modulation of spinal nociception and pain: The impact of predictable noxious stimulation. *Pain, 126*(1–3), 221–233.

Rimke, H. (2000). Governing citizens through self-help literature. *Cultural Studies, 14*(1), 61–78.

Robertson, A. F. (2001). *Greed: Gut feelings, growth and history*. Cambridge: Polity Press.

Roenneberg, T., Kuehnle, T., Juda, M., Kantermann, T., Allebrandt, K., Gordijn, M., & Merrow, M. (2007). Epidemiology of the human circadian clock. *Sleep Medicine Reviews, 11*, 429–438.

Romme, M., & Escher, S. (Eds.). (1993). *Accepting voices*. London: Mind Publications.

Romme, M., Escher, S., Dillon, J., Corstens, D., & Morris, M. (2009). *Living with voices: 50 stories of recovery*. Ross-on-Wye: PCCS Books.

Rose, N. (1985). *The psychological complex*. London: Routledge.

Rose, S. (1997). *Lifelines: Life beyond the gene*. Oxford: Oxford University Press.

Rose, N., & Abi-Rachid, J. (2013). *Neuro*. Princeton, NJ: Princeton University Press.

Rosenbaum, P., & Valsiner, J. (2011). The un-making of a method: From rating scales to the study of psychological processes. *Theory and Psychology, 21*(1), 47–65.

Rosenstock, I. M. (1974). Historical origins of the health belief model. *Health Education & Behavior, 2*(4), 328–335.

Ross, C. E., Mirowsky, J., & Pribesh, S. (2001). Powerlessness and the amplification of threat: Neighbourhood disadvantage, disorder and mistrust. *American Sociological Review, 66*, 568–591.

Ruiz, J., Hutchinson, J., & Terrill, A. (2008). For better and worse: Social influences on coronary heart disease risk. *Social and Personality Psychology Compass, 2*(3), 1400–1414.

Ruthrof, H. (1997). *Semantics and the body*. Toronto: University of Toronto Press.

Sampson, E. E. (1983). *Justice and the critique of pure psychology*. New York: Plenum Press.

Sanders, T. (2005). It's just acting: Sex workers' strategies for capitalising on sexuality. *Gender, Work and Organisation, 12*(4), 319–342.

Santiago-Delefosse, M. (2012). Deconstructing the notion of 'belief' in psychology: Commentary on 'Beyond belief'. *Journal of Health Psychology, 17*(7), 974–976.

Saunders, L. (2015). The challenge of CFS/ME in primary care. In C. Ward (Ed.), *Meanings of ME: Interpersonal and Social Dimensions of Chronic Fatigue*. London: Palgrave.

Sayce, L. (1998). Stigma, discrimination and social exclusion: What's in a word? *Journal of Mental Health, 7*, 331–343.

Scarry, E. (1985). *The body in pain*. Oxford: Oxford University Press.

Schacter, S., & Singer, J. (1962). Cognitive, social and physiological determinants of emotional state. *Psychological Review, 69*, 379–399.

Scheff, T. (2000). Review: Michael Billig 'Freudian repression'. *Human Relations, 53*(12), 1603–1610.

Scheff, T. (2003). Male emotions/relations and violence: A case study. *Human Relations, 56*(6), 727–749.

Scheff, T. (2011). Social – emotional origins of violence: A theory of multiple killing. *Aggression and Violent Behavior, 16*(6), 453–460.

Scheff, T. (2013). A social/emotional theory of 'mental illness'. *International Journal of Social Psychiatry, 59*(1), 87–92.

Scheff, T., & Fearon, D. S. (2004). Cognition and emotion? The dead end in self-esteem research. *Journal for the Theory of Social Behaviour, 34*(1), 73–90.

Scheff, T., & Mahlendorf, U. (1988). Emotion and false consciousness: The analysis of an incident from Werther. *Theory, Culture & Society, 5*(1), 57–80.

Scherer, K. R. (2009a). The dynamic architecture of emotion: Evidence for the component process model. *Cognition and Emotion, 23*(7), 1307–1351.

Scherer, K. R. (2009b). Emotions are emergent processes: They require a dynamic computational architecture. *Philosophical Transactions of the Royal Society B: Biological Sciences, 364*(1535), 3459–3474.

Scully, P., Quinn, J. F., Morgan, M. G., Kinsella, A., O'Callaghan, E., Owens, J. M., & Waddington, J. L. (2002). First-episode schizophrenia, bipolar disorder and other psychoses in a rural Irish catchment area: Incidence and gender in the Cavan – Monaghan study at 5 years. *British Journal of Psychiatry Suppl*, 181 (suppl 43), s3–s9.

Seale, C. (2005). New directions for critical internet health studies: Representing cancer experience on the web. *Sociology of Health and Illness, 27*(4), 515–540.

Sedgewick, E., & Frank, A. (1995). *Shame and it's sisters: A Silvan Tompkins reader*. Durham, NC: Duke University Press.

Seeman, T., Dubin, L., & Seeman, M. (2003). Religiosity/spirituality and health: A critical review of the evidence for biological pathways. *American Psychologist, 58*(1), 53–63.

Segal, B. (1988). *Alcoholism etiology and treatment: Issues for theory and practice*. New York: Haworth Press.

Sharpe, M. (1998). Cognitive behaviour therapy for chronic fatigue syndrome: Efficacy and implications. *American Journal of Medicine, 105*, 104s–109s.

Sharpe, M., Hawton, K., Clements, A., & Cowen, P. J. (1997). Increased brain serotonin function in men with chronic fatigue syndrome. *British Medical Journal, 315*, 164–165.

Sharpley, M. S., Hutchinson, G., & Murray, R. M. (2001). Understanding the excess of psychosis among the African-Carribean population in England. Review of current hypotheses. *British Journal of Psychiatry Suppl, 178* (suppl. 40), 60s–68s.

Sheets-Johnstone, M. (1999). *The primacy of movement.* Amsterdam: John Benjamin.

Shilling, C. (2003). *The body and social theory* (2nd ed.). London: Sage Publications.

Shotter, J. (1989). Social accountability and the social construction of 'you'. In J. Shotter & K. J. Gergen (Eds.), *Texts of Identity* (pp. 133–151). London: Sage Publications.

Shotter, J. (1993a). *Conversational realities: Constructing life through language.* London: Sage Publications.

Shotter, J. (1993b). *Cultural politics of everyday life.* Buckingham: Open University Press.

Shotter, J. (1993c). Bakhtin and Vygotsky: Internalisation as a boundary phenomenon. *New Ideas in Psychology, 11*, 379–390.

Shusterman, R. (Ed.). (1999). *Bourdieu: A critical reader.* Oxford: Blackwell.

Shweder, R. A. (2004). Deconstructing the emotions for the sake of comparative research. In A. Manstead, N. Frijda & A. Fischer (Eds.), *Feelings and Emotions: The Amsterdam Symposium* (pp. 81–97). Cambridge: Cambridge University Press.

Siddique, H. (2014, 2 April). World's first computational psychiatry centre opens in London. *The Guardian.* Retrieved from http://www.theguardian.com/science/2014/apr/02/worlds-first-computational-psychiatry-centre-london.

Silagy, C., Mant, D., Fowler, G., & Lodge, M. (1994). Meta-analysis on efficacy of nicotine replacement therapies in smoking cessation. *The Lancet, 343*(8890), 139–142.

Simmons, J. P., Nelson, L. D., & Simonsohn, U. (2011). False-positive psychology. *Psychological Science, 22*(11), 1359–1366.

Skeggs, B. (2004). *Class, self and culture.* London: Routledge.

Sloan, R., & Bagiella, E. (2002). Claims about religious involvement and health outcome. *Annals of Behavioural Medicine, 24*, 14–21.

Sloan, R., Bagiella, E., & Powell, T. (1999). Religion, spirituality and medicine. *The Lancet, 353*, 664–667.

Smail, D. J. (1984). *Illusion and reality: The meaning of anxiety.* London: J. M. Dent.

Smail, D. J. (1987). *Taking care: An alternative to therapy.* London: J. M. Dent.

Smail, D. J. (1993). *The origins of unhappiness.* London: Constable.

Smail, D. J. (2005). *Power, interest and psychology: Elements of a social materialist understanding of distress.* Ross-On-Wye: PCCS Books.

Smith, C. (2007). Why Christianity works: An emotions-focused phenomenological account. *Sociology of Religion, 68*(2), 165–178.

Snell, W. E., Gum, S., Shuck, R. L., Mosley, J. A., & Kite, T. L. (1995). The clinical anger scale: Preliminary reliability and validity. *Journal of Clinical Psychology, 51*(2), 215–226.

Sokolov, A. N. (1975). *Inner speech and thought*: Springer Science & Business.

Stam, H. (1998). The body's psychology and psychology's body. In H. Stam (Ed.), *The Body and Psychology* (pp. 1–12). London: Sage Publications.

Stearns, P. (2008). Fear and history. *Historein, 8*, 17–28.

Stein, M., & Rauch, S. (2008). Do syndromes matter (DSM)? *Depression and Anxiety, 25*, 273.

Stenner, P., & Stainton-Rogers, R. (2004). Q methodology and qualiquantology: The example of discriminating between emotions. In Z. Todd, B. Nerlich, S. McKeown & D. Clarke (Eds.), *Mixing Methods in Psychology: The Integration of Qualitative and Quantitative Methods in Theory and Practice* (pp. 101–120). Hove: Psychology Press.

Stephenson, N., & Papadopoulos, D. (2007). *Analysing everyday experience: Social research and political change*. London: Palgrave Macmillan.

Stepper, S., & Strack, F. (1993). Proprioceptive determinants of emotional and nonemotional feelings. *Journal of Personality and Social Psychology, 64*(2), 211–220.

Stern, D. (1985). *The interpersonal world of the infant: A view from psychoanalysis and developmental psychology*. New York: Basic Books.

Stevanovic, M., & Perakyla, A. (2014). Three orders in the organization of human action: On the interface between knowledge, power, and emotion in interaction and social relations. *Language in Society, 43*, 185–207.

Stich, S. (1983). *From folk psychology to cognitive science: The case against belief*. Cambridge, MA: MIT Press.

Stokkan, K.-A., Yamazaki, S., Tei, H., Sakaki, Y., & Menaker, M. (2001). Entrainment of the circadian clock in the liver by feeding. *Science, 291*(5503), 490–493.

Stuckler, D., & Basu, S. (2013). *The body economic: Why austerity kills*. London: Allen Lane.

Sullivan, G., & Strongman, K. (2003). Vacillating and mixed emotions: A conceptual-discursive perspective on contemporary emotion and cognitive appraisal theories through examples of pride. *Journal for the Theory of Social Behaviour, 33*, 203–226.

Sutherland, S. (1996). *The international dictionary of psychology (Revised Edition)*. London: Crossroad Classic.

Tallis, R. (2009). Neurotrash. *New Humanist, 124*(6). Retrieved from http://newhumanist.org.uk/2172/neurotrash.

The Free Association. (2011). *Moments of excess: Movements, protest and everyday life*. Oakland, CA: PM Press.

Thomas-Maclean, R., & Stoppard, J. (2004). Physicians's constructions of depression: Inside/outside the boundaries of medicalisation. *Health, 8*(3), 275–293.

Throop, C. J., & Murphy, K. M. (2002). Bourdieu and phenomenology: A critical assessment. *Anthropological Theory, 2*(2), 185–207.

Tietze, C., Lemkau, P., Cooper, M., & Burgess, E. (1941). Schizophrenia, manic-depressive psychosis and social-economic status. *American Journal of Sociology, 47*(2), 167–175.

Timimi, S., & Taylor, E. (2004). ADHD is best understood as a cultural construct. *British Journal of Psychiatry, 184*, 8–9.

Tolman, C. (1994). *Psychology, society, subjectivity: An introduction to German critical psychology*. London: Routledge.

Tom, G., Pettersen, P., Lau, T., Burton, T., & Cook, J. (1991). The role of overt head movement in the formation of affect. *Basic and Applied Social Psychology, 12,* 281–289.

Tracy, S. (2010). Qualitative quality: Eight 'Big-tent' criteria for excellent qualitative research. *Qualitative Inquiry, 16*(10), 837–851.

Trafimow, D., Sheeran, P., Conner, M., & Finlay, K. (2002). Evidence that perceived behavioural control is a multidimensional construct: Perceived control and perceived difficulty. *British Journal of Social Psychology, 41,* 101–121.

Trevarthen, C., & Aitken, J. (2001). Infant intersubjectivity: Research, theory, and clinical applications. *Journal of Child Psychology and Psychiatry, 42*(1), 3–48.

Triandis, H. C., Bontempo, R., Betancourt, H., Bond, M., Leung, K., Brenes, A., Georgas, J., Hui, C. H., Marin, G., Setiadi, B., Sinha, Jai B. P., Verma, J., Spangenberg, J., Touzard, H., & Montmollin, G. (1986). The measurement of the etic aspects of individualism and collectivism across cultures. *Australian Journal of Psychology, 38*(3), 257–267.

Trower, P., & Chadwick, P. (1995). Pathways to defence of the self: A theory of two types of paranoia. *Clinical Psychology: Science and Practice, 2,* 263–277.

Tsai, J., Miao, F., & Seppala, E. (2007). Good feelings in Christianity and Buddhism: Religious differences in ideal affect. *Personality and Social Psychology Bulletin, 33*(3), 409–421.

Tucker, I. (2004). 'Stories' of chronic fatigue syndrome: An exploratory discursive psychological analysis. *Qualitative Research in Psychology, 1,* 153–167.

Turner, J. (2000). *On the origins of human emotions.* Stanford: Stanford University Press.

Tyler, S., Hertel, P., McCallum, M., & Ellis, H. (1979). Cognitive effort and memory. *Journal of Experimental Psychology: Human Learning and Memory, 5*(6), 607–617.

Tyrer, P. (2001). The case for cothymia: Mixed anxiety and depression as a single diagnosis. *British Journal of Psychiatry, 179,* 191–193.

Van Damme, S., Crombez, G., Houdenhove, B. v., Mariman, A., & Michielsen, W. (2006). Well-being in patients with chronic fatigue syndrome: The role of acceptance. *Journal of Psychosomatic Research, 61,* 595–599.

van der Veer, R., & Valsiner, J. (1991). *Understanding Vygotsky: A quest for synthesis.* Oxford: Blackwells.

Vangeli, E., & West, R. (2012). Transition towards a 'non-smoker' identity following smoking cessation: An interpretative phenomenological analysis. *British Journal of Health Psychology, 17*(1), 171–184.

Vanwesenbeeck, I. (2005). Burnout among female indoor sex workers. *Archives of Sexual Behavior, 34*(6), 627–639.

Vetlesen, A. (2011). Atrocities. A case of suppressing emotions or of acting them out? *Passions in Context, II*(1), 36–66.

Voronov, M., & Singer, J. A. (2002). The myth of individualism-collectivism: A critical review. *The Journal of Social Psychology, 142*(4), 461–480.

Vygotsky, L. S. (1962). *Thought and language* (E. Hanfmann & G. Vakar, Trans.). Cambridge, MA: M.I.T. Press.

Vygotsky, L. S. (1978). *Mind in society: The development of higher psychological processes.* Cambridge, MA: Harvard University Press.

Ward, C. (2015). The said and the unsaid: Ambivalence in CFS/ME. In C. Ward (Ed.), *Meanings of ME: Interpersonal and Social Dimensions of Chronic Fatigue.* London: Palgrave.

Wendell, S. (1996). *The rejected body: Feminist philosophical reflections on disability.* London: Routledge.

Werner, A., & Malterud, K. (2003). It is hard work behaving as a credible patient: Encounters between women with chronic pain and their doctors. *Social Science & Medicine, 57*(8), 1409–1419.

Werner, S., Malaspina, D., & Rabinowitz, J. (2007). Socioeconomic status at birth Is associated with risk of schizophrenia: Population-based multilevel study. *Schizophrenia Bulletin, 33*(6), 1373–1378.

Wertsch, J. (1991). *Voices of the mind: A sociocultural approach to mediated action.* Hemel Hempstead: Harvester Wheatsheaf.

Wertz, F. (2011). The qualitative revolution and psychology: Science, politics, and ethics. *The Humanistic Psychologist, 39*, 77–104.

Westermeyer, J. (1989). Paranoid symptoms and disorders among 100 Hmong refugees: A longitudinal study. *Acta-Psychiatrica-Scandinavica, 80*, 47–59.

Wetherell, M. (1995). Romantic discourse and feminist analysis: Interrogating investment, power and desire. In C. Kitzinger & S. Wilkinson (Eds.), *Feminism and Discourse: Psychological Perspectives* (pp. 128–144). London: Sage Publications.

Wetherell, M. (2012). *Affect and emotion: A new social science understanding.* London: Sage.

Wetherell, M. (2015). Tears, bubbles and disappointment – new approaches for the analysis of affective-discursive practices: A commentary on 'Researching the psychosocial'. *Qualitative Research in Psychology, 12*(1), 83–90.

Whitehead, A. (1927). *Process and reality.* New York: The Free Press.

Whitehead, L. (2006). Toward a trajectory of identity reconstruction in chronic fatigue syndrome/myalgic encephalitis: A longitudinal qualitative study. *International Journal of Nursing Studies, 43*(8), 1023–1031.

Wierzbicka, A. (1999). Emotional universals. *Language Design, 2*, 23–69.

Willig, C. (1995). 'I wouldn't have married the guy if i'd have to do that': Heterosexual adults' constructions of condom use and their implications for sexual practice. *Journal of Community & Applied Social Psychology, 5*(2), 75–87.

Willig, C. (2001). *Introducing qualitative research in psychology.* Buckingham: Open University Press.

Willig, C., & Stainton-Rogers, W. (Eds.). (2007). *The sage handbook of qualitative research in psychology.* London: Sage Publications.

Wilson, E. A. (1999). Critical/cognition. *Annual Review of Critical Psychology, 1*, 136–149.

Wilson, E. A. (2004). *Psychosomatic: Feminism and the neurological body.* Durham/London: Duke University Press.

Wilson, M. (2002). Six views of embodied cognition. *Psychonomic Bulletin & Review, 9*(4), 625–636.

Woolgar, S., & Pawluch, D. (1985). Ontological gerrymandering: The anatomy of social problems explanations. *Social Problems, 32*(3), 45–61.

Wortham, S. (2001). Review of Michael Billig, Freudian repression. *Discourse Studies, 3*(2), 253–255.

Wright, C., Fischer, H., Whalen, P., McInerney, S., Shin, L., & Rauch, S. (2001). Differential prefrontal cortex and amygdala habituation to repeatedly presented emotional stimuli. *Neuroreport, 12*(2), 379–383.

Wyer, R. (1974). *Cognitive organisation and change: An information processing approach.* Hillsdale, NJ: Earlbaum.

Young, I. M. (1990). *Throwing like a girl and other essays in feminist philosophy and social theory*. Bloomington, IN: Indiana University Press.

Young, I. M. (1998). Throwing like a girl: Twenty years later. In D. Welton (Ed.), *Body and Flesh: A Philosophical Reader*. Oxford: Blackwell.

Zajonc, R. B. (1980). Feeling and thinking: Preferences need no inferences. *American Psychologist, 35*(2), 151–175.

Zajonc, R. B. (1984). On the primacy of affect. *American Psychologist, 39*(2), 117–123.

Ziebland, S., Chapple, A., Dumelow, C., Evans, J., Prinjha, S., & Rozmovits, L. (2004). How the internet affects patients' experience of cancer. *British Medical Journal, 328*, 564–569.

# Index

Printed and bound by CPI Group (UK) Ltd, Croydon, CR0 4YY